HAMER

A CRITICAL LOOK AT HEALTHCARE

MARK HANLEY

HAMER

A CRITICAL LOOK AT HEALTHCARE

First Edition May 2018

© 2018 Mark Hanley
All rights reserved

ISBN 978-1-7320877-0-5

Companion Website
http://www.acriticallookat.com

This book is dedicated to all those who will not be satisfied with anything but the truth regarding their health. I will not claim to have found it, as to me, this is a journey, not a destination, but I can claim to sense a dead end road when I'm on one. After decades of traveling, I feel I must speak up, having found more than my share of cul-de-sacs, and a single, more than promising alternative route, that to me just feels right. To keep quiet, to bite my tongue, in the face of what to me were monumental discoveries, is unconscionable. I must in good faith share this with anyone who will listen.

RGH • RIP

The secret of medicine is to distract the patient while Nature heals itself.

Voltaire

Legal Disclaimer

The information in this book is intended to augment your knowledge of existing modes of healthcare, not replace your personal relationship with your doctor. I have collated existing knowledge for your convenience and added my opinion of this knowledge; it should never be construed as a diagnosis, treatment, prescription, advice or cure for any disease. Always consult a qualified medical professional for specific health concerns; do not rely on this material for medical treatment.

Full disclosure: I am an engineer by training, an occasional patient by fate; I am NOT a doctor. I am not rendering medical advice or services to the individual reader and am therefore not liable or responsible for any loss, damage, anguish or distress allegedly arising from any information or suggestion in this book. I approach the task of writing this book as a medical layman. Because of this, I must, and will gladly, rely heavily on the words of professional healthcare sources themselves to assess the state of their services, followed, of course, by my own opinions of such.

I make what to me is a reasonable assumption, that these medical professionals are honestly depicting their disciplines in their publications (web, books, articles). Although I seldom quote from them directly, I have provided endnotes (see *Endnote Instructions* chapter) to all relevant material. I rarely name specific medical organizations, as that information is largely irrelevant to my arguments. I am not affiliated with any of the medical paradigms or organizations or linked material explored in this book. I have no control over their content, and consequently, assume no responsibility for them. Most links are web pages that naturally contain more material than the context of my endnote would suggest. As I also have no control over that, I therefore also assume no responsibility for that extraneous content.

Contents

iv Legal Disclaimer

1   Introduction

DEFINITIONS

8   The Problem

11 The Cure For Disease

16 The Brain Controls All Cells

19 The Subconscious Brain

21 The Germ

24 The Virus

31 The Somatid

35 The Mainstream Solution

39 The Ancient Solutions

41 The Royal Solution

43 The Alternative Solutions

45 The Maverick Solution

59 The Medicine

62 The Epidemic

67 The Placebo

HEALTHCARE

72 Allergies

77 Bones And Cartilage

87   Brain

95   Cancer

114 Central Nervous System

120 Heart

130 Kidneys And Bladder

135 Liver And Gallbladder

144 Lungs

152 Mental Illness

161 Pancreas

168 Skin

CONCLUSION

178 Patient Hat

182 Status Quo

185 GNM

190 Extras

194 Final Thoughts

. . .

196 Reference

198 Appendix

202 Index

211 Endnote Instructions

212 Endnotes

v

Diagrams

27 Polio incidences plotted against pesticide production

32 Somatid cycle (credit Dr. Gaston Naessens)

47 German New Medicine SBS progression

61 Affect of medicine on CA and PCL phases

97 7 year generic cancer survival chart

98 5 vs 7 year generic cancer survival chart

Introduction

The topic of this book is healthcare. In a broader sense though, I am just attempting to communicate. I, like everyone, have a worldview, a set of conclusions based on what I call my knowledge base, which is nothing more than data I have gathered throughout my life. I label every piece of data in my knowledge base as either true, false, or unknown. These labels are not carved in stone, as new data often results in a reevaluation of old assessments. I contend, that you, being a reasonable person, would arrive at my conclusions if you had my knowledge base, as I would arrive at yours were our roles reversed. If you are dissatisfied with your opinion of health care in the West, or are curious about this topic in general and are open to new ideas, then it is my hope you will find something of value in these pages. I approach this study from an American vantage point but am pretty sure my analysis holds for Western medicine in general.

There will be those who take offense to my questioning this part of society. After all, who am I? Perhaps they will feel that so important a topic should be left to trained medical professionals (of which I am not), and from a medical practice standpoint, I agree with them, but there are many different healing paradigms. One cannot simply leave health to doctors, as they are not all of one mind, even within a given modality. They're a little bit like analog clocks in that regard: if you have one, you always know the time, if you have two, you seldom do. Doctors can and do disagree wildly with one another, especially on health issues attached to dismal prognoses. Within the wide net that encompasses all doctors,

Introduction

you will find a smorgasbord of opinions concerning health. Which opinion will you trust? Since there are millions of doctors one could consult, the strategy, *let the doctor decide*, begs the question, *which doctor?*

To answer that, one must first answer the question: *Which medical paradigm is best for my particular health concern?* Then finally: *Which doctor in that paradigm do I trust with my health?* As daunting as that task may be, I submit that the answers can only come from you; after all, it is your health. You are the only one who must travel that road. Once that final question is answered, the details of navigating your way back to health are best discovered leveraging the skill of that doctor. Their role in your journey is a function of their particular medical expertise. If I consult a surgeon about a medical problem, there is a good chance they will offer surgery as the solution. If instead, I turn to a homeopath, there is a good chance that I will instead receive a recommendation to place several little white sugar balls under my tongue. Who can say which of these doctors is right for your particular medical issue? It is your body, your journey, the choice is properly yours (or your guardian should your society not recognize your ability to decide for yourself). To choose wisely, you need information, which I attempt to augment with this book.

To aid in your decision, I offer the following observation. All medical paradigms are based on core theories, sets of ideas that attempt to explain health and sickness. These foundational concepts attain axiom status, are no longer questioned, to allow the science to advance. They are assumed to be fact, though, in all likelihood they are not. These assumptions become the basis of all theories within the paradigm that follow, and will inevitably face challenges, as those who proposed the axioms are not omniscient. How a given paradigm deals with those objections reveals much about the integrity of its adherents. I contend that there are but two ways to deal with such challenges: the political way, in which observed fact is subservient to agenda, and the honest way, in which agenda yields to observed fact. It is perhaps an idealistic way of looking at the issue, but in your search to regain your health, I submit that the paradigm most beneficial to your goal is the one that most embraces the honest way. There exists a direct correlation between the extent to which facts are massaged in a given medical paradigm to fit axiom and the danger such distortions pose to your health. Understand, every medical (for that matter, just plain every scientific) theory proposed by man is, by definition, wrong. The question is only, to what extent is it wrong? The nature of this inquiry will necessarily resolve to either a preponderance of the evidence or its lack. Your glass half-full or half-empty preferences will lead you to embrace the paradigm that either proves the most correct or the least incorrect to your judgment.

In 1957, an American social psychologist, Leon Festinger, proposed his theory of Cognitive Dissonance (CD)[1], in which he describes a powerful urge to maintain a consistent worldview even in the face of facts that contradict one's knowledge base. It explains why otherwise reasonable people cannot accept even plain truths when faced with evidence that severely threatens their psychological harmony. It reveals why some would knowingly embrace falsehoods rather than reassess their conclusions. CD provides fertile breeding grounds for all manner of Rube Goldberg-esque rationalizations. Such a reaction, while perhaps deserving of compassion, does not bode well for building a solid foundation of health and healthcare. These topics demand the truth, or at least as close as we can get. They insist on no small dose of critical thinking, as Nature is seemingly indifferent to suffering, caring not a whit about anyone's feelings, their worldview, their CD, or just how badly she's about to discredit their preferred medical paradigm. Embrace her path in this regard as best you can to avoid pain, suffering and death; be indifferent to it or ignore or reject it at your peril.

Introduction

This book is as much an opportunity for me to gather my thoughts on health and healthcare, as it is for me to share my research. I draw many conclusions, and can only assume I have arrived near the truth. It is up to each reader to decide how you'll tally my score. It is my sincere wish that through this book, you will be able to add useful data to your knowledge base to further solidify your thoughts on healthcare, and hopefully thereby, lead a healthier and happier life.

Healthcare as a percentage of GDP[2] (2015 data) has reached 10% worldwide, with expenditures in the United States accounting for roughly 1 of every 6 (17%) dollars spent. Given that the world's 2016 GDP was in the neighborhood of $120 trillion[3] (all $ references in this book are United States dollars), humans spent roughly $12 trillion on health care in 2016. Americans accounted for $3.2 trillion of that amount, or $10,000 per person per year, which is approximately the average global per capita income.

It seems prudent, in the face of such enormous expenditures, to perform periodic, independent audits on such an essential part of society. I intend to do just that with this book. Were I a doctor, much, if not all, of the independence would be lost, relegating the effort, at least in some part, to an exercise in propaganda. Sweeping questions spring to mind: Is the end goal of the dominant medical paradigms even health? Are the popular methods currently in use sympathetic to that goal? In our quest to reach this goal, which roads are being ignored or suppressed? Are status quo concepts of what health and disease are even correct? Where are we on this journey? What, if any, medical paradigm makes the most sense? These are personal questions that demand personal answers; I am unaware of a universal solution to any such problem. We may come to the same conclusions, but the stakes are far too high not to draw your own.

Introduction

Mainstream or conventional medicine is the primary beneficiary of this vast ongoing financial expenditure. It must, therefore, receive the bulk of my scrutiny, as millions of people still suffer and die annually from the very conditions this money is, and historically has been, intended to alleviate.

I hope to provide answers as best I can to these questions. I should also like to stimulate a conversation in your head as to what approach you will take to regain your health should you lose it. Ideally, you would decide while you are well. Choosing say a cancer treatment, after you have been diagnosed with cancer, is a bit like picking up a *How To Swim* book while drowning. At that point, time is often of the essence. This and the emotional trauma of the event may force you to defer that choice to someone you trust. Regardless of your choice, it is always wise to seek professional medical advice before proceeding with any strategy to regain or maintain your health.

One of the benefits to me as the author of this book is that this is, by its nature, not a dialog. All I can do is lay out my case. I cannot consider your input to the subject, as you are not giving it while I write. Given the nature of this topic, I expect such would be lively and given my hopes for a sizable audience, probably overwhelming. So, it is ideal for me to simply share, and for you to decide what, if any of this, to embrace. We will all at some point in our lives, be interested in how illness and healthcare work, and so we share a vested interest in trying to get as close as we can to the truth, as this topic is objective, so not swayed by conjecture.

This work makes heavy use of endnotes, the reading of which is greatly simplified by my companion website (see the *Endnote Instructions* section). The endnotes are optional but highly recommended reading.

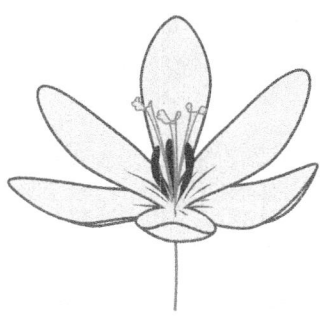

Definitions

The Problem

With 7+ billion people living on this planet, it is no surprise that there exist an enormous variety of health problems and a very thick catalog of ideas of how to deal with them. There is an old saying: a healthy person has many wishes, a sick person only one. Well, wishing to be well again, hinges heavily on what methods you invoke to regain your health. Simply wishing is rarely successful. Usually one must also act, if only to stop doing what you did that first compromised your health. So the question becomes: how will you act?

That all depends I suppose on what is wrong with you; just how your health is compromised. The first logical step is to answer that question; what is the cause of your trouble? You may not find the answer, or you may not have time to look before you treat symptoms, or the cause may be obvious or absent, but unless you determine cause, your chance to correct the problem, or at least not repeat it, is relegated to dumb luck. I for one, am more than uncomfortable with trusting to such. Doing so will likely see you spending a lot of time, money, and discomfort merely managing symptoms, and praying to whoever you think will listen for relief.

To determine cause, it helps to have a broad understanding of what can go wrong with you. I use the following (admittedly non-comprehensive) list:

A. **Small trauma:** Cuts, scrapes, bruises, etc.
B. **Malnutrition:** Scurvy, rickets, marasmus, dehydration, etc.
C. **Large trauma:** Knife wound, gunshot wound, dog bite, car accident, broken bone, etc.
D. **Poison:** Snakebite, spider bite, drugs, chemicals, radiation, rancid or spoiled food, unclean water, etc.
E. **Parasites:** Tapeworm, intestinal fluke, hookworm, etc.
F. **Disease:** Heart disease, cancer, respiratory disease, Alzheimer's, diabetes, mental illness, etc.

Of this list, many people will deal with A themselves at first, resorting to professional help only upon complications. This is merely my observation of common behavior, not a recommendation, a disclaimer that applies to the rest of the items on this list as well. Determining the cause of a cut or scrape will let you know whether the wound is clean, or whether you should consider steps other than cleaning and dressing the wound.

B is often handled like A, if the symptoms are recognized. The related adverse effects to one's health from B are likely another matter, best treated by medical professionals. A common reaction to health insults of this nature is to add the missing nutrients to your diet, which presupposes you know what they are.

C is handled quite competently by modern hospitals and doctors. It falls into squarely into the category of **NOT** do-it-yourself. The protocols of the professionals in this field have noticeably improved over the years, and will no doubt continue to do so. As I argue in the next chapter, causes for these injuries are often irrelevant.

Definitions

For D, antitoxins presuppose the toxin is known. Administering snake anti-venom to a victim of lead poisoning is at best pointless. Rancid oils are rejected by the human body as the gastrointestinal tract recoils in violent spasms, leaving the victim resembling nothing if not a double barrel bolus cannon. Spoiled food and dirty water can have a similar effect, though the offending poisons are most often the byproducts of microbial decay. Likewise, it is no secret that our food chain is subject to all manner of chemicals and artificial genetic modifications. Putting aside the benefits to production and profit, just how does their presence affect our health? Again, any health insults in this category, like C, are best left to medical professionals.

E is effectively handled by a combination of herbs and protocols[4] or prescription drugs. Any adverse effects, like B, are best left to medical professionals. Knowing cause here will hopefully lead to prevention.

That leaves F, an extensive category of compromised health that consumes the lion's share of health care expenditures. From my layman's vantage, it appears the least understood and therefore, in my opinion, most in need of an audit. Cancer, heart disease, lung issues, stroke and Alzheimer's top the leading causes of death list in my country and are all members of this category. I will leave the discussion of cause in these illnesses to later chapters. **Note**: this category of health issues is the primary focus of this book.

Whichever route is taken to regain health, the buck will stop with you. You are the one that will make this journey. You are the one who will experience the pain, the discomfort, the despair, and hopefully, the relief and elation should your health return. No one can do this for you. Others can only help or hinder. It is up to you to embrace the former and reject the latter. Knowledge is your friend in this choice. How you use it is up to you.

The Cure For Disease

Mainstream, well actually most, medical terminology includes the cornerstone words *disease* and *cure*. The first is intended to define a state of less than optimal health, and the second, an external substance or procedure it is hoped will restore this lost optimal health.

Disease, or illness, or sickness, are words that imply something is wrong with you, with your health; perhaps even that you are a danger to others. For some reason, there are stigmas attached to some diseases (mental illness, leprosy, AIDS, etc.) while others are more likely to elicit sympathy. In my view, all these reactions, positive and negative, are born of ignorance and fear. If it were possible to alleviate the ignorance, would that be enough to dispel such emotions? I recommend keeping this question close while reading this book.

Very often disease is seen as an attack, from an external source; a foe to be vanquished, conveniently by the application of a medicine, a cure. In this way of thinking, Nature has failed or been overcome, necessitating the assistance of a doctor, who by expertly introducing medications to the patient or performing procedures on them, expedites their return to health. I remind the reader that I am only considering the health concerns of category F, as defined on the previous page.

While this is one way of looking at the issue, I suggest it is not the only way, and in fact, hope to provide you food for thought that it is not even the best way. There is an old saying that if you do nothing for a

Definitions

cold, it will be gone in a week, if you take medicine, you'll be well again in seven days. I am not equating all disease with a cold; I am suggesting that it is your body that will do all the healing. A doctor may alleviate symptoms, thereby making a patient feel better, less sick, but any *cure* will come from Nature. Your body will right itself, or it won't (a fact I contend is greatly influenced by knowledge). Acute situations in this category may result from prolonged neglect, often through ignorance on the part of the patient, and require a doctor to intercede, but you are not sick because you lack a particular medicine coursing through your veins, or because you have not experienced a specific medical procedure.

A *cure* in this regard, defined as above as an external substance or procedure intended to restore optimal health, is nonsense. It suggests that the body is incapable of repairing itself and that outside help must be sought if health is to be restored. As doctors are a human phenomenon, and a relatively recent one at that, the first time any creature fell seriously ill would be its last. By now, there would be no life whatsoever on this planet. Understand that defining a cure as an external substance or procedure intended to alleviate uncomfortable symptoms while a patient regains their health is an altogether different proposition. Take, for example, a pain reliever. Such a drug can clearly lessen discomfort, ushering welcome sleep or rest, but it is Nature that will do the healing, the curing, with or without the pain relief. How does this fundamental conclusion differ from the direction of most medical research?

Anxiety and fear are ever-present in society today concerning health. I suggest that this is due, in large part, to ignorance. Health care is chiefly the province of professionals. An overwhelming majority of people immediately turn to doctors when sick, having little clue as to why they are sick, and even less of what to do about it, other than, of course, to defer to a professional. While consulting a medical professional about health concerns is a good idea, dumping everything in their lap and hoping they can deal with it is not. It is at best unfair to the doctor. Health in this scenario frequently becomes a spectator sport, where the patient passively sits on the sidelines hoping for a positive outcome while the doctor makes all the decisions, and takes all the actions. Since another person, even a trained medical professional, cannot make your body heal itself, is it any wonder then that the mythical idea of a cure has taken root? You get what you pay for indeed.

It is arrogant to hold an opinion such as, *There is no cure*, as it ironically assumes omniscience, which none of us, not even doctors, possess. Appending the phrase *using our methods*, or, *of which I am aware*, would right the statement, at the expense of the doctor's authority, so it should come as no surprise that it is seldom heard. To me, such pretense is directly related, however unconsciously, to a dismissal of Nature's role in health. When it is held by a medical professional and shared with a trusting, hopeful patient, the resulting realization can be devastating. After all, if the expert is throwing up their hands, what chance does the patient have? Hopelessness and doom are not welcome on anyone's road to recovery.

I suppose that an apt metaphor for this book is a treasure hunt. The treasure I seek is cause; answers to the questions: what causes this or that illness? To me, these are fundamental questions, the answers to which drive all rational efforts to overcome disease and return to health. Until recently, my answers to these questions at best failed to convince me. I don't believe I will ever have THE answers (if such exist), but personally, I need to be close enough to be comfortable. To ignore the questions is to resign yourself solely to fate. Perhaps Nature will see you through to health; perhaps she won't. How lucky do you feel? Relying exclusively on Nature is the only path, as best we can tell, that all life other than humans (OK, and their extensions – pets and livestock) must travel. For this, they appear to have a primal instinct that guides them, and to which they comply, a faculty we seem to lack. Is our's overwhelmed by the constant chatter of our minds?

I for one, am not satisfied with resigning myself to fate. Nor am I content with trusting my health care to medical professionals who cannot answer the question of cause to my satisfaction. Name one situation where addressing a problem while remaining ignorant of its cause ends in actual success. If your car tire wears prematurely, was it a bad tire, or is your suspension at fault? If it's the suspension, and you simply replace the tire (treat the symptom), you can expect the new tire to fail again quickly. If a relationship is broken, and you ignore cause to focus on symptoms, whatever fix you apply will be temporary. For example: if your friend is irritated because you continuously interrupt, telling a funny joke might momentarily change their mood, but unless you address the cause, unless you stop interrupting, you can expect their grumpy mood to quickly resurface and the relationship to further deteriorate. Likewise, if you suffer from a health problem, and don't address the cause, you are simply rolling the dice, hoping Nature figures it out and corrects the problem. Moreover, if you address anything other than that cause, you may actually interfere with what Nature is doing to fix the problem. If you suffer a fever, and you take a medicine to reduce it, it seems prudent to ask yourself why it was there. Was the fever your body's way of dealing with another problem, and in reducing it, have you interrupted or interfered with a repair perhaps more critical to your health? What are the consequences of that action? I am not suggesting that you ignore a fever; I am proposing that all of these issues can be mitigated or even eliminated if you have a solid understanding of cause.

My acid test for whether a medical modality has a rational explanation of cause is the common cold, something virtually everyone on this planet can relate to firsthand, and from what I can tell, is as rampant as ever, even in tropical climates where it is rarely, if ever, cold. If your preferred doctor can explain what a cold is, to your satisfaction (not merely how to treat symptoms), how and why it happens, without contradictions or exceptions, then I suggest you listen. If they can't unambiguously explain such a seemingly simple malady, what confidence will you find in their guidance should the stakes get serious?

It is not for me to process an explanation of cause for you. Everyone must do this for themselves. Your knowledge base will drive your conclusions. I ask this question of cause throughout Section 2 (Healthcare) of this book. The data may surprise you.

There is one paradigm which I will explore which studies subconscious reactions to personal events. It is more than just a traditional medical paradigm as it illuminates Nature's survival strategies, of which departure from, and return to health are but parts. While this may sound perhaps both brazen and out of place in a book auditing healthcare, it is neither. The insight that led to this discovery was born of fate and cancer. With it, causal ignorance (and subsequent fear) of disease, can be overcome by scrutinizing the first law of Nature – survival. With it, the myriad emotions surrounding disease are rightfully shifted from the patient, to the events that eventually led to disease. With this insight, human judgement of any aberration of bodily function (in category F) is relegated to the absurd, as none of us are even remotely qualified to question Nature's methods. Much more on this paradigm to follow.

The Brain Controls All Cells

The field of embryology[5] informs us that the first organs to develop in vertebrates are the brain and spinal cord, i.e. the nervous system. From there, bud-like clusters form at the end of nerves. As the fetus grows, these buds become your vital organs, your heart, liver, kidneys, etc. In this way, the central nervous system connects all parts of the body to the brain. These connections (brain relays) allow the brain to monitor and control all parts of the body. This communication extends to the cellular level, either directly through electrical (nervous) stimulation or indirectly through chemical stimulation.

It stands to reason that it is in the best interest of the organism that all of its parts behave as one cohesive whole. We surely would have died out as a species if the eyes observed a predator but the legs were unaware, or if one leg panicked and went left while the other panicked right, or if one muscle cell contracted while its neighbor relaxed. The brain receives sensory input, and controls and coordinates the desired reaction. Much of this effort is subconscious; I was unaware until recently just how much.

Chickens slaughtered by decapitation, often fly away headless (so by inference brainless), only to plummet to the earth dead a short distance later. This flight is undoubtedly a complicated action, coordinated without an actual brain, implying a brain-like function somewhere within the rest of the chicken. Since an intact chicken does possess a brain organ, I can only conclude that this backup brain, wherever it is, is an evolutionary holdover. Surely when the original organ is present, the backup is idle?

Vines like cucumber, grape, ivy all move their branches in circular motions while *climbing*, stopping once they make contact with something they can latch onto, and yet, I know of no cucumber, grape or ivy *brain*. This observation though leads me to conclude that there is a brain like function in their cells too, as the circular motion, and the subsequent wrapping around the object they encounter appears to be a coordinated effort among many cells. Is this evidence of an evolutionary cell brain? Perhaps as an organism evolves in size and complexity, Nature sees fit to move complex functions into a dedicated organ. The kidneys process water, the lungs gas, the heart circulates blood, and the brain is control central.

It seems that the brain can exercise that control to the DNA level[6], which really, given its control over all other aspects of the body should not come as too great a surprise. In addition to controlling body cells, it appears that the brain even controls bacteria present in the body. A chiropractor by the name of Robert H. Walker wrote a book in 1951 titled *Functional Processes Of Disease*. In it, he reports on an experiment whereby 12 rabbits were inoculated with an extra-lethal dose of virulent septic staphylococci bacteria in their abdominal cavity. The researchers then severed the rabbit's vagus nerves below the diaphragm, in effect blinding the rabbit's brain relays that communicate via that nerve, and observed the results. Seven of the twelve rabbits succumbed from the experiment, but the remaining five recovered. Furthermore it was noted that the expected inflammation, which would normally spread throughout the abdomen, remained localized in all the rabbits. Did the seven die because of the bacteria, or the general shock of the experiment? Unfortunately, the report does not say. Rabbits are known to be highly stress sensitive. Stories of rabbits dying from fright alone

Definitions

are not uncommon. All we can glean for certain from this report is that just under half of the test subjects escaped certain death.

So it seems that the brain even exercises control over infection, over germs, as the bacteria apparently behave one way with a working nerve connection to the brain, and another way without. How does mainstream medical science account for this?

The Subconscious Brain

Your brain will try its best to keep you alive, keep you safe. Your subconscious mind will act if your conscious mind will not, or cannot. What I mean by that, is that just because you may be consciously unable to react to a situation, that does not mean that nothing is being done to assist you. The primary goal of Nature, unsurprisingly, seems to be to survival. This goal is accomplished in many ways: sexual desire, hunger, thirst, fear. The desire to live is overwhelmingly strong.

A mother lifts a car off of a child, straining or even tearing ligaments, tendons, and muscles in her arms, shoulders, legs and back, but not feeling the pain until the child is safe. This example involves a mother's child, an extension of herself biologically. She doesn't think; she acts — immediately. If she thought about it, brought the situation into her conscious mind, she would most certainly conclude she couldn't lift the car.

I remember a tornado event in my past. I was watching the bad weather outside when I witnessed the roof of my neighbor's house vanish in the blink of an eye. I froze. The next thing I remember was flying down the stairs to the basement as fast as my feet could carry me as the air was sucked out of my house. I don't remember consciously heading there. It was as if, knowing my conscious mind was paralyzed by fear, my subconscious took over and hurled me down to safety.

Definitions

Another example from my past involved a wasp in a classroom in high school. I was zoning out as the teacher lectured about some topic in History. I was in a trance of sorts, twirling my pencil in random patterns between my fingers. I became aware of a wasp on a window in the room. As I looked at it, it flew towards me. I remember thinking, it's going to sting me, but there was no panic. As it neared my hand, I flicked the pencil across its flight path in a perfectly timed arc, cutting it in two. Watching its two halves spinning in their death throes on the floor, I snapped out of my trance, as my buddy whispered, "How did you do that?" I honestly had no idea. Today, I chalk it up to another small example of my subconscious mind protecting me.

What else will the subconscious mind do to keep you from harm besides animating your muscles? Will it command an increase or decrease in cells to boost or retard function temporarily? Will it quickly grow more alveoli in response to a perceived need for more oxygen? Will it strengthen bone in response to perceived weakness? Will it increase blood flow to the heart in response to a territorial challenge by ulcerating the interior of arteries thereby widening them? Will it retain water in response to perceived isolation by limiting water excretion from the kidneys? We will explore these possibilities and more in later chapters.

The Germ

No single person has had a greater impact on health care in the West than Louis Pasteur. His advocacy of germs being the cause of disease is the bedrock of mainstream western medical thought.

Louis Pasteur (1822-1895) was a French chemist and biologist. He spent a great deal of time studying fermented liquids under a microscope. Seeking to understand why they sometimes soured, Pasteur noticed the presence of microbial forms (germs) and became convinced that they were responsible for the spoilage. Since he found no evidence of these germs in the unfermented liquid, he concluded that they were in the air, floating all around us; that they sought out the liquid, attacked it so to speak, and caused its deterioration. This eureka moment is the modern birth of the Germ Theory of disease.

While this is one explanation, one theory, it is not the only one. A countryman and contemporary of Pasteur, Antoine Béchamp, championed a different theory to explain the same facts. He proposed that diseased terrain attracted germs as scavengers of a sort. He noticed, however barely, tiny energetic entities in liquids whose function he did not fully understand. He named them microzymas (tiny ferments) as they enable fermentation. They are a vital component of the Terrain Theory of disease; a concept expanded on in a later chapter entitled *The Somatid*.

Definitions

Germ Theory proposes that germs are external to the host, that they wander in from the outside and then attack. If the host is weak, the germs may overwhelm and multiply. If the host is healthy, their immune system will overcome the invaders. It imagines war at a microscopic level. It has given rise to the pharmaceutical industry which is largely responsible for producing the weapons for this war.

It is logical to assume that germs *eat* and that a primary reason for engaging with another species is to do just that. They don't have mouths with teeth like people, but they must take in nutrients to live. J. R. R. Tolkien was referring to midges in *The Lord Of The Rings* when he had Sam ask: "What do they live on when they can't get hobbit?" Surely the same can be asked of germs.

If these microscopic entities can live on other sources of food, why risk the hostile environment of the human (or any animal's) immune system? If they can't, they should have either all starved to death a long time ago, or be present in large numbers in every human host on this planet, a proposition, which according to the best mainstream medical testing, is demonstrably false.

How is feeding on human flesh biologically advantageous to a germ? Surely it is not a conscious effort by germs to throw caution to the wind and mix things up a little by attacking the relatively sophisticated defenses of humans for a meal? Nor does it seem likely that they are just toying with us, making life miserable for the fun of it, kind of like what cats do sometimes to mice. Perhaps there is more to the germ narrative than Pasteur or even Béchamp, imagined?

The two theories, Germ and Terrain, are incompatible with one another. Western medicine has bet the farm, and your health, on the former. To me, however, the question of which is more correct is unresolved, as disease is still a major global problem. It seems to me that it would not hurt to direct a little bit of money and effort at the Terrain Theory. After all, Rudolph Virchow[7], the father of pathology is quoted as saying: "If I could live my life over again, I would devote it to proving that germs seek their natural habitat—diseased tissue—rather than being the cause of the diseased tissue; e.g., mosquitoes seek the stagnant water, but do not cause the pool to become stagnant." Pasteur himself is rumored to have recanted on his deathbed, referring to Pasteur's contemporary and friend, the physiologist Claude Bernard (1813-1878), saying: "Bernard is right; the microbe is nothing, the terrain is everything."[8] Surely if these two champions of the Germ Theory expressed doubts, it is in our best interests to heed their concerns.

For a significant clue to the answer to this question of whether germs cause disease, consider the sad case of Masha and Dasha[9], Siamese twins born in Russia in 1950 who were the subject of medical experimentation and research. The girls had individual upper torsos but shared the lower half of their body, as well as a circulatory system. Here is the part to ponder: they did not get the same diseases. As children one twin got measles, the other did not. One would *catch a cold*; the other would not. Whatever medical theory you embrace should account for this. Remember, agenda should yield to fact, not the other way around. Sweeping inconvenient facts under the rug is a signature tactic of proponents of the political way.

The Virus

An axiom in mainstream medicine is that germs cause disease. It is a proposition that is not questioned. If a Western mainstream doctor finds an infection where bacteria (or other visible microbes) are not present, then some other pathogen is suspect. Enter the virus.

Dr. Robert Koch was a celebrated physician and pioneering microbiologist, who in 1890 published a set of rules for determining pathology known today as Koch's postulates:

1. The germ must always be present, in every case of the disease, but not in healthy subjects.
2. The germ must be isolated from a diseased host and grown in pure culture.
3. This cultured germ must cause the same disease when injected into a healthy host.
4. The germ must then in turn be isolated from the formerly healthy host and be identical to the original germ.

His medical contributions were held in such high regard that the German government named their central scientific institution in the field of biomedicine in his honor: the Robert Koch Institute (RKI). Dr. Koch's postulates present a very logical progression indeed within the Germ Theory framework, albeit one with several holes, or diseases that don't fit the pattern. Yet historically, Koch's postulates were embraced by mainstream medicine, and it is my understanding that postulate 3 is still revered as truth. Notice that a critical requirement (postulate 2) involves isolating the suspected pathogen. To isolate means to separate unto itself, to obtain a pure sample. Ignoring the validity of these postulates when applied to bacteria, do they hold true for viruses?

Stefan Lanka[10] is a German Ph.D. who was studying microbiology at university just as the acquired immune deficiency syndrome (AIDS) scare was ramping up in Europe in the mid-1980s. My understanding is that while researching AIDS, he contacted RKI for information on human immunodeficiency virus (HIV), a key suspect in AIDS, including any photos of the isolated virus (taken with an electron microscope), as Koch's second postulate demands. He received a package, but none of the images were of isolated viruses. There were artist conceptions (drawings), images of blood constituents, etc., but none of verified (original document reference) isolated HIV viruses. Later, he requested the same for other viruses (measles, polio, smallpox, etc.). As before, he received many images, but none of verified isolated viruses.

After decades of futility in isolating any virus implicated in causing disease in humans, in 2011, Dr. Lanka offered a prize of €100,000 to anyone who could provide scientific proof of a virus responsible for measles. Dr. David Bardens attempted to claim the award by supplying Dr. Lanka with published medical studies. Dr. Lanka rejected this evidence, and Dr. Bardens sued, winning an initial judgment. The case[11] was appealed, and in 2016, the decision was overturned, ruling in favor of Dr. Lanka.

The court apparently opined that the publications in question do not rise to the level of proving the existence of a virus responsible for measles; trial experts cited lack of control experiments in the publications. That does not mean that the measles virus doesn't exist, it simply means that their existence (in isolation) has yet to be proved, at least to the satisfaction of the German High Court. It also does not mean that a measles virus is not responsible for causing measles, but without isolation, the Koch sequence stalls on the first step. Proof that a virus is responsible for measles first requires isolation, which despite the apparent low hanging fruit of the substantial prize, has apparently yet to be achieved. Of curious note: apparently, RKI claims to have made just such studies of the measles virus, but to date, has not published its findings. We are left to wonder why.

The implications of this are enormous. If viruses have not been isolated, have not been proven to be causal agents in disease, let alone been proven to even exist, then what exactly are the active ingredients in vaccines? We know what the inactive ingredients are: thimerosal (a compound of mercury), aluminum, formaldehyde, others. Many are toxic to humans and are reportedly included to weaken the virus or spur a greater immune response. What are the ramifications of bypassing the body's natural defenses and injecting known toxins directly into the bloodstream? Since infants are the prime target of vaccines (49 injections from 14 vaccines, from in utero to age six years),[12] exactly how does such repeated exposure to these toxins affect the most vulnerable among us? Vaccine damage awards in the US alone have exceeded $3.7 billion since 1989,[13] which I accept as proof that some have been negatively affected, as the average award exceeds $650,000. A vaccine is supposed to boost immunity by introducing a human immune system to a weakened or even dead virus, or in some cases, parts of a virus. To do so would obviously entail first isolating said virus, a critical requirement apparently as yet unmet. Indeed, the procedures for isolating viruses range from filtering based on physical size (super-small mesh filters), to specific antibody affinity chemistry, resulting in a soup of ridiculously tiny things, many of which are unknown. My earlier mental image of a vaccine lab technician plucking distinct viruses from a known, controlled culture, to include in a vaccine was apparently

The Virus

fantasy. If the virus part of the vaccine is then suspect, the only thing we know for sure is that we have strict laws[14] that mandate repeatedly dosing babies with poisons.

The poster child for vaccine efficacy is the polio vaccine. Examine the following chart to decide for yourself if polio was defeated by the Salk and Sabin vaccines. It should be clear from the graph that reports of polio were already dropping hard when Dr. Salk introduced his vaccine. Incidences continued to plummet after that, but at seemingly identical rates, leading me to question if his vaccine had any effect. Dr. Sabin introduced his vaccine to a US population largely devoid of polio, so it is difficult to determine its efficacy from US data. Superimposed on the same graph[15] is US production of a class of persistent pesticide (DDT, BHC, lead and calcium arsenates). Consider that polio adversely affects the central nervous system, as do these pesticides, and note which graph leads the other. Was polio the result of pesticide poisoning?

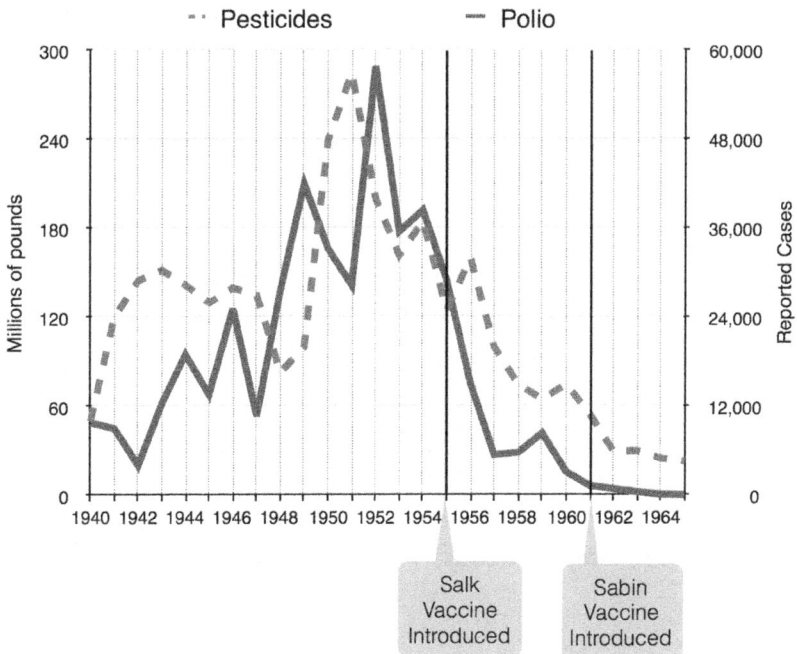

Definitions

One obvious conclusion from all this is that the claim that viruses cause disease is but one part of the Germ Theory of disease, not the Germ Fact of disease. Facts are the world's data. Theories are sets of ideas that attempt to explain facts. That people fall ill is a fact. That microscopic pathogens are the cause of such trouble is a theory. To be considered science, any theory must be falsifiable (the proposition that ideas that better explain the facts are always waiting to be discovered), or it is dogma. Is the Germ Theory of disease false? By definition, it must be, or it is a religion, and then why bother with proof; why bother with all this talk of science? Assuming it is science, the question is then: to what extent is it false?

As if this coffin needs another nail, Janine Roberts, an investigative journalist, published a book in 2008, called *Fear of the Invisible*. In it, she discusses an article,[16] published online by the Centers for Disease Control and Prevention entitled *Isolation and Identification of Measles Virus in Cell Culture, Revised Nov 29, 2001*. The article discusses the very topic for which Dr. Lanka offered his prize. From the title, you would think someone in government would have just sent Dr. Lanka the article, and reduced the burden of the US taxpayer by the amount of his prize. Once I read Ms. Roberts' summation of the process, it is clear to me why that never happened.

The current procedure[17] is apparently little changed from the 2001 article. What follows is my understanding of the current instructions.

- Obtain a specimen from a measles patient (urine, nasal mucous, saliva). It is assumed that the sample contains the measles virus.
- Obtain Vero/hSLAM cells (kidney epithelial cells isolated from African green monkeys). Epstein-Barr virus transformed marmoset B lymphoblastoid cells (B95a) were previously used.[18] (link section 5.4.1)

- Obtain fetal bovine serum (FBS), which is blood from cow fetuses from which all red blood cells have been removed.
- Obtain trypsin, a digestive enzyme for dissolving protein, from pig pancreases. Ignore any non-enzyme pig-part constituents that may have escaped filtration and are present in the enzyme solution.

1. Prepare a DMEM culture for hosting Vero/hSLAM cells by adding antibiotics (penicillin, streptomycin, and geneticin).
2. Wash the monkey cells in a bath of trypsin, which will begin to dissolve them, as kidneys are largely protein, and further, kidney epithelial cells are bound together with proteins.
3. Thoroughly mix cells from step 2 into the prepared culture from step 1, to which 10% FBS has been added.
4. Incubate for 24 hours at body temperature.
5. Add to this mix, more culture from step 1 and 1 ml of the patient's specimen. Incubate for 1 hour at body temperature.
6. Observe cells under a microscope to see if the sample show signs of infection (floating or rounding of Vero cells). The implication is that the monkey cells are now infected with measles virus, though no actual measles virus has been detected.
7. Continue this observation, adding trypsin at intervals until observed Vero/hSLAM cell damage reaches 50% or more.
8. If this occurs, scrape the cells (and whatever else comes with) off the top. You now have a viable viral stock, ready for use in vaccines. I guess they should add pig trypsin and stale antibiotics to the list of possible toxins in the measles vaccine.

No control culture (same process sans specimen) to compare, no actual detection of the virus, only inference, no telltale signs of measles (the culture cells are monkey kidney, whereas measles manifests on the skin), no assurances that the specimen or the pig-sourced trypsin or the monkey kidney cells or the bovine fetus serum did not contain other microbes or tiny unknowns, which may now be present in the measles

Definitions

vaccine stock. This (along with the previously mentioned inactive ingredients) is what is injected first into babies.

I fail to see why a theory which,

1. often cannot meet its own reasonable guidelines,
2. has failed to defend itself against an axiomatic challenge in a court of law,
3. is supposedly used to create vaccines which in turn are burdened by stacks of admittedly anecdotal evidence showing harm, especially to young children,
4. is the basis for a preventive apparently created by following a recipe which appears to require the suspension of logic and reason to understand,

is defended so rigorously as fact. Perhaps it is perceived as a better than nothing solution to an admittedly frightening reality. Is it wise, given these many open questions, to concentrate the overwhelming bulk of research efforts on this path? Does not this uncertainty warrant casting a wide net into side streams in our search for answers? Viewed in this light, the hounding and persecution of those who are already exploring those alternative avenues seems at best unjustified.

The Somatid

Typical optical microscopes have limits to their magnification and resolution. They can magnify roughly 1,000-2,000 times and resolve to 2,000 angstroms. Despite these limitations, they have a significant advantage, as they allow the scientist to observe living things, quite useful when your subject is microbiology.

Electron microscopes have much higher magnification and resolving powers, along the lines of 10,000,000 times magnification and 0.5 angstroms resolution. These powerful views into the truly tiny come at a cost. The energy directed for viewing is fatal to living tissue.

Royal Raymond Rife[19] was an inventor, who in the late 1920s created what he called The Universal Microscope. It was an optical microscope with the ability to magnify to 60,000 times. Rife's microscope design (dark field microscopy) used resonance to self-illuminate his subject material. He discovered that this technique, if not carefully applied, would disturbingly cause his subject material to shake themselves to pieces. He proceeded to compile a list of these mortal oscillatory rates (MOR), which included entries for BX and BY, pathogens he suspected of causing cancer. His resonant antibiotic method was crushed using litigation when Rife reportedly refused to share his discovery[20] with Morris Fishbein, the first head of the American Medical Association (AMA).

Definitions

Roughly ten years later, a French inventor, Gaston Naessens, invented a similarly powerful optical microscope which he named the Somatoscope. It is capable of 30,000 times magnification with a resolution of 150 angstroms.

While observing blood specimens under high magnification with his Somatoscope, Dr. Naessens saw swarms of tiny, vibrant entities swimming in blood, as well as in the sap of plants. They were few and lethargic in samples from sickly specimens. He named them somatids,[21] hence the name of his microscope. They are what Pasteur's contemporary Béchamp had previously named microzymas, but could not fully describe, due to their minute size and the limits of his conventional optical microscope. Experimenting with the blood cultures, Dr. Naessens was able to induce profound physical changes in the somatids by gently changing (heat, etc.) their medium.

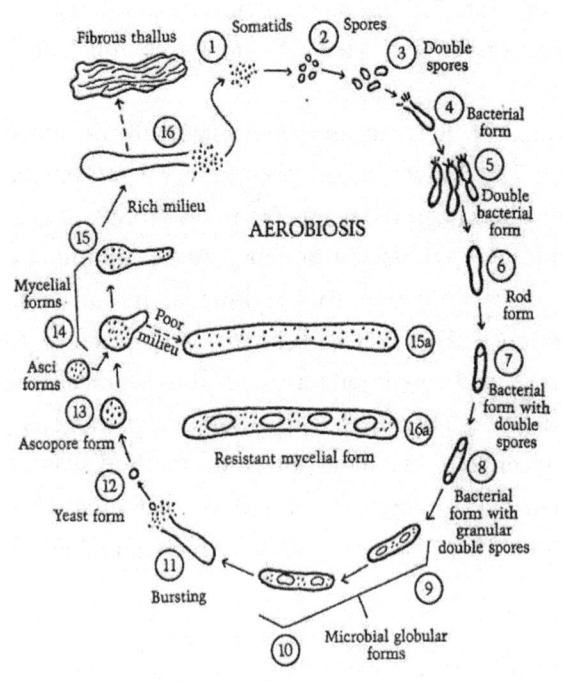

16 state somatid cycle (Image courtesy of CERBE Distribution, Inc.)

I can't help but wonder if fever contributes to this phenomenon in the body. Dr. Naessens cataloged this cycle of change, identifying somatids as pleomorphic, that is, being able to assume multiple forms, including bacteria. Note that he did not observe a virus form.

Dr. Naessens' work with somatids provides an answer to a previous mystery: from where do bacteria and yeast present in the human body come? We have assumed that some are foreign invaders introduced by what we breathe or ingest, or encounter via wounds; that some are beneficial while others are harmful.

Somatidian Orthobiology, as Dr. Naessens calls this study, shows an alternate explanation, one with a profound implication. If some (or all) microbes are outgrowths of a normal part of our bodies, indeed of all living things, then it is logical to assume that they are there for our benefit, as all parts of any life form naturally serve a biologically meaningful, positive purpose.

Are then microbes present in infection, there to help us? Are we mistaking their presence as malignant? We have observed all too many times that infections can overwhelm and even kill a patient. Dr. Naessens describes an "inner biological protection gate", a boundary (separating states 3 and 4) between normal and pathogenic states of these pleomorphic forms. What controls that transition? We note with alarm that our defense against germs has become increasingly less effective with time, as witnessed by the panic surrounding methicillin-resistant staphylococcus aureus (MRSA) in hospitals. The standard theory is that the germs must be evolving to counter the antibiotics. If the antibiotic does not kill all the germs present, those left would be naturally resistant, and left to replicate. While that is certainly a possible explanation, it is not the only credible one.

Definitions

What if we require these forms for our health, in ways not commonly understood? What if their controller, which in humans would seem to be our brain, is actively manipulating them in an effort to sidestep the antibiotic? If that is so, our goal of controlling microbes with antibiotics is likely doomed, as Nature is ever so much more clever in pursuit of her prime directive than any medical researcher. Can these homegrown bacteria harm us, and if so, how, or is it just external bacteria that we need to fear? If we are not to die of infection, what other strategies to regain our health are we not understanding?

The author Daniel P. Reid, in his book *The Tao of Health, Sex, & Longevity*, reported on a curious phenomenon.[22] The ashes of the cremated bodies of a select few Buddhist and Taoist monks, who in life achieved the highest levels of their meditative discipline, can contain thousands of tiny, luminous, indestructible nuggets. Indeed, the ashes of a Taiwanese monk who died in the 1950s reportedly contained over 10,000 of these ssu-lee-dze (relic seeds). Allegedly not found in other people (could it be that they are just too small, and therefore not noticed?), these *nuggets* are impervious to hammer blows and knife cuts, are somewhat opaque and are reported to glow. Mr. Reid explains that skilled adepts collect a "Golden Elixir" in their lower abdominal energy centers over a lifetime of meditation. During cremation, relic seeds are formed from the burning of this elixir.

Contrast that to Christopher Bird's description of somatids in his book *The Trial and Persecution of Gaston Naessens*.[23] In it, he tells of the seemingly indestructible nature of somatids, having been shown to be unaffected by heating to 200° C, exposure to 50,000 rems of radiation, emersion in strong acids, and finally, failed attempts to cut them with a diamond blade. Could it be that Golden Elixir is a concentrated form of this fundamental element of life? How exactly does meditation affect them? What other secrets can somatids yield about life?

The Mainstream Solution

Western or conventional medicine is an umbrella catchphrase that encompasses a dominant percentage of healthcare professionals in the West. Here in the United States of America, practitioners of Western medicine are primarily found in hospitals and clinics where they characteristically use surgery, drugs, and radiation to treat symptoms of disease.[24] Another word for this type of medicine is allopathy.[25] A network of universities specializing in medical education organized through the Association of American Medical Colleges (AAMC), and after graduation, a network of physicians, the American Medical Association (AMA), support this medical paradigm.

Allopathy is the basis for successful emergency room (ER) medicine. What is common in many ER cases is clear cause. What I mean by that is that often, either the cause of the injury is no longer present or is readily identifiable. A few examples should clarify my position:

1. **A person was hit by a car:** The cause of their injuries is blunt force trauma, caused by a vehicle that is no longer present. The ER physicians need not concern themselves with cause, and are free to treat the symptoms of the collision.
2. **A person falls while skiing and ruptures her ACL:** The ligament is in 2 pieces. Left alone, it will not heal by itself. The current procedure is to replace the ACL with a hamstring, taken either from the patient, or a cadaver, and attach it surgically to the bone where the torn ligament once

was. The cause is water under the bridge to the surgeon, and irrelevant to the repair.
3. **A person is a victim of gunfire:** If the cause (bullet or fragments) is still present, removal is necessary. Once the bullet is gone, addressing the symptoms by cleaning and closing the wound and repairing internal damage (in this simple example) is indicated. Again there is no mystery as to cause, and again, it is irrelevant to treatment (assuming the bullet is not radioactive or poisoned).

It is evident that many complications can arise from ER medicine. I am not in any way trying to say it is simple, quite the contrary. There are patients whose symptoms do not clearly indicate what is wrong with their health, and yet are in dire need of medical intervention to save their lives; not every case has clear cause. ER doctors do however often have the luxury, and indeed the necessity, of ignoring cause and proceeding straight to symptom treatment. I suppose you could seek alternative care for health problems such as these, but in many if not most of these cases, you would probably be referred posthaste right back to the ER. They have the most and best resources to deal with such insults to your health.

The problem, as I see it, is in thinking that the same methods and practices that work so well for ER medicine are applicable, and indeed preferable, for all types of health issues. Leveraging the enormous expense of an emergency room hospital by attempting to make it the hub of a one-size-fits-all solution to health care would seem to be a ready-made solution, but as economically attractive as that may be to hospital administrators, I have serious doubts that it represents the best solution for the consumer of healthcare services. A simple observation that allopathic medicine is the default health system in the West and that the leading cause of death in the West is not natural causes, but a plethora of prematurely fatal diseases from category F (cancer, diabetes, etc.) makes me question the efficacy of this approach to healthcare. Medical authorities report [26] that 70% of global deaths (37% in low-income countries to 88% in high-income countries) are caused by non-communicable diseases (NCDs). Globally, apply those percentages to 55+ million deaths annually to arrive at a figure of just under 40 million people dead each year from diseases that allopathy has targeted for a century with mountains of money. We all have to die of something as nobody lives forever, but category F deaths (roughly equivalent to NCDs) are seldom easy, and I, for one, would rather not take the hard road if I have a choice.

Technology has always led Western medicine to ever more precise estimates of what is wrong with a person's health. X-rays allowed the physician to look inside the body without surgery. Later computed tomography (CT) scans employed computers to merge a series of x-rays to create cross-sectional or even 3-D images of the body. Magnetic resonance imaging (MRI) exposes the body to a strong magnetic field that causes specific atomic nuclei to emit radio frequencies that are then used to create alternative images to x-rays. Positron emission tomography (PET) scans use radioactive dyes injected into the bloodstream to illuminate a patient from within so that sophisticated sensors can precisely map soft tissue.

All of this to identify disease, and yet very little clarity on why it should exist in the first place. Western medicine is very good at answering what, and less good at answering why. Unfortunately, knowing why is a crucial first step in understanding how best to respond to disease. Allopathic doctors see germs in a disease site and conclude germs caused the disease. They notice that the DNA of cells in some diseases differs from the same cells in healthy people and conclude that the altered DNA is causing the problem. They observe that people living

Definitions

with certain environmental factors have statistically higher rates of certain diseases and conclude that those factors are somehow causal in their disease.

Perhaps, but there are certainly other ways of looking at the problem. Finding flies at a garbage dump fools nobody into thinking that the flies caused the garbage. Conventional wisdom holds that DNA is static and that changes occur due to random events, such as exposure to radiation. A classic DNA related disease is sickle cell anemia, wherein red blood cells with this altered DNA take on a different shape. It turns out, this adaption protects against malaria (a tropical parasitic disease), at the expense of oxygen transporting efficiency, so it's a tradeoff, the lesser of two evils. I suppose this could be a random mutation, but then why is it almost exclusively found in people (and their descendants) chronically exposed to malaria? Could it be that this is not a random mutation, but rather a deliberate natural one – directed by the (subconscious) brain? Are other DNA related diseases also a Scylla and Charybdis choice?

The use of statistics in determining cause is fraught with pitfalls. They are used to try to make sense of something where not enough data is known. As the founder of nuclear physics, Sir Ernest Rutherford noted: "if your experiment needs statistics, you ought to have done a better experiment." Indeed, an extreme example of this trap would be to check the sock color of cancer patients and then falsely conclude that wearing blue socks carried with it a higher risk of cancer.

All of this is to say that there is more than one way to interpret the facts we see; there are many theories of health and disease. In this book, I explore several other ways to interpret the data. I implore you to decide what makes the best sense to you.

The Ancient Solutions

Medical traditions that extend millennia into the past serve fully half of the world's population. Two of the largest and most established of these Eastern traditions are Traditional Chinese Medicine (TCM), and Ayurveda.

Neither historically view disease as an attack by microscopic enemies or some genetic flaw, but rather as an imbalance in a body's energy. Subsequently, they approach healing in a very different way than the Western mainstream. Their primary focus has been, and still is, on restoring balance to that energy.

TCM is thousands of years old. Three classic texts codifying medical principles that are still in use today were written during the Han Dynasty, roughly 2,000 years ago. They put to print ideas that took millennia to develop. They are *The Yellow Emperor's Classic of Internal Medicine, Shen Nung's Pharmacopeia,* and *Discussion of Fevers.* According to TCM, when yin and yang[27] are balanced, there is health; otherwise, there is illness. Therefore, TCM practitioners will seek to either tonify a lack of yin or yang, or disperse an excess thereof.

Ayurveda is a medical paradigm developed in India thousands of years ago. Its core principles are that mind and body are one and that nothing can heal the body better than the mind. According to Ayurveda, life force manifests as three distinct energies or doshas[28]: Vata, Pitta, and Kapha. Life is animated by a unique combination of these three

Definitions

energies. Health ensues when they are balanced, illness when they are not.

Both of these medical systems have served billions upon billions of people with excellent results. For me, they get much closer than the Western mainstream in identifying cause but personally stop short of a satisfying answer. Both see disease as an imbalance in body energies. Both identify the cause of disease as either an excess or lack of a particular energy, and seek to counter this deviation from the optimum to restore balance and therefore health.

And yet neither fully addresses why a particular energy should be imbalanced, pointing to stress and diet as major culprits. There are plenty of examples of stressed or malnourished people with no symptoms of illness, just as, in critiquing mainstream medical wisdom, there are plenty of people who smoke and drink and live to a ripe old age. So too, there are people who display symptoms of AIDS or other infectious diseases yet test negative for the suspect microbe, as well as people who test positive and yet show no signs of the disease.

The Mainstream and Ancient solutions are the primary medical answers for the majority of people on this planet. Is there another theory of health that nails the cause issue so that a truly effective solution to poor health can be discovered?

The Royal Solution

Homeopathy is a field of medicine created in 1796 by Samuel Hahnemann. It is applicable in categories A, C (post-recovery) and F outlined in a previous chapter titled *The Problem*. German royalty and through them, most famously, British royalty, have enthusiastically supported homeopathy almost since its inception.[29] It operates from a principle of *like cures like*. By trial and error, homeopathy claims that if a substance causes a specific set of symptoms in an otherwise well person, then a minute amount of that substance in a person suffering from those symptoms will stimulate a healing response in their body.

Homeopathic remedies are made by diluting substances in water to the point where there may not be a single molecule of the original substance left in the final solution. The solution is then commonly combined with sugar (lactose or sucrose) and pressed into tiny balls to be placed under the tongue for rapid sublingual absorption. Rare is the objection made by children to taking this form of medicine.

Critics cite the dilution of the remedies as proof that homeopathy is nothing more than a placebo, ignoring the observation that homeopathy seems to work in babies and animals, neither of which would have an understanding of placebos or expectations of a remedy. There is also a marked lack of side effects, unlike its pharmaceutical counterparts.

Research aimed at establishing efficacy and toxicity has admittedly not been anywhere near as thorough as allopathic testing, due to

Definitions

funding limitations (the current homeopathic market is much smaller than the patent medicine space), and the inherent lack of risk due to the extremely low doses of what allopaths would deem as the active ingredient. What testing there is, is generally that of the randomized control trial (RCT), where double blind placebo controlled test subjects are used, just as in allopathy, with intriguingly similar results.

A British homeopathic organization[30] revealed that peer-reviewed journals had published 104 placebo-controlled RCTs involving homeopathic remedies for 61 medical conditions through 2014. Of these RCTs, 54% proved inconclusive, while 41% indicated that the medicine had a positive effect on the patients health, with the remaining 5% indicating a negative effect. These data compare favorably to an admittedly far larger sample size of conventional medicine placebo-controlled RCTs from 1,016 such peer-reviewed journals, wherein 49% of the remedies tested proved inconclusive, 44% proved positive, and 7% proved negative. So, 41% to 44% positive, 5% to 7% neutral, and 54% to 49% non-conclusive. To me that's six of one, half a dozen of the other. Statistical stability grows with sample size, and 104 tests, though not trivial, is less than ideal. Still, I feel it is realistic to place a fair measure of confidence in the results of this comparison.

Homeopaths (doctors of homeopathy) treat either symptoms or the whole patient. This second approach is referred to as constitutional homeopathy. Symptom treatment is indicated when a condition exists that is acute, where the symptoms are known to disappear as the body heals itself eventually. Homeopathic constitutionals are recommended for chronic health problems, ones that don't seem to heal.

Compared to allopathic remedies, or pharmaceuticals, the price of homeopathic remedies are exceedingly low, making them an attractive alternative to anyone seeking to curb the expense of health care.

The Alternative Solutions

With global spending on health care running roughly $12 trillion annually, there are obviously a large number of doctors providing services. As I have argued earlier, imposing a one size fits all solution to health care seems at best sub-optimal. So, in addition to the mainstream health solutions, there are hundreds of so-called alternative healthcare solutions. They exist for a number of reasons, among which is the fact that despite truly incomprehensible amounts of money being spent on the mainstream approach, a major cause of death is that people get sick and prematurely die. They don't just die of old age in their sleep; they too often die from complications of their illness or its treatment. In fact, iatrogenic (doctor-induced) death trails only heart disease and cancer[31] in areas of the world where allopathic health care is the norm. So some people quite naturally look to solutions outside of the mainstream (even if their insurance doesn't cover the costs), a most irrational reaction had the mainstream all, or even most, of the answers.

In addition to the solutions outlined in the previous two chapters, principal players in alternative health solutions[32] are summarized below:

Chiropractic[33] is a branch of health care that focuses on skeletal and muscular manipulations to remedy certain health concerns. Complaints such as back, neck, and joint pain, as well as headaches are most often addressed.

Definitions

Naturopathic[34] medicine is a collection of modern, traditional, scientific and empirical medical methods that focus on encouraging natural healing processes to regain health. Disease prevention is a large part of the Naturopathic regimen.

There are easily hundreds of more methods and modalities that fall under this *alternative* umbrella. Please refer to the link in the endnote above (32) for more information. It is difficult to generalize about alternative health solutions given the size of the list, but mostly, the cost is far less than the mainstream approach. Alternative diagnostic methods include iridology, foot and ear reflexology, tongue, skin and pulse testing, none of which require expensive high-tech equipment.

Dr. Fereydoon Batmanghelidj[35] championed the absolute least expensive alternative approach to medicine I have ever found. Dr. B, as he was affectionately known, was born in Iran, and studied medicine in Great Britain. After the overthrow of the Shah of Iran in the Iranian revolution in 1979, Dr. B was confined to prison for two years for political reasons. During that time, he had no access to any of the medical supplies he was accustomed to in his practice. Still, there were demands of his help, as stress among the prisoners was understandably very high. He prescribed the only thing he had access to one day to a prisoner with severe stomach pains, water. Within minutes, the prisoner felt relief. Dr. B continued to witness the curative powers of just water during his confinement and continued this research after his release. He used his conclusion for the title of one of his books: *You're Not Sick, You're Thirsty*. Lots of clean water and a pinch of salt (to replace electrolytes eliminated in the accompanying frequent urination) were his medicine, used to great success. It really doesn't get any less expensive than that.

The Maverick Solution

German New Medicine[36] (GNM) is the name given to a set of five biological laws or observations discovered by Dr. Ryke Geerd Hamer (1935-2017). It is an understanding of health radically unlike any of the others presented in this book. What follows is my admittedly incomplete understanding of Dr. Hamer's work, which I discovered in 2014. I believe I have a firm grasp on the core of GNM; specific details are for me an ongoing education. A relative lack of English texts on this subject is, in part, the reason for my writing. I have read all the books listed in the reference section in the back of this book, taken online GNM courses, watched many videos both in German and English, and scoured the web for hundreds of GNM articles. I share my understanding only in the hope that it will pique your interest in GNM, and recommend that you avail yourself of the reference section to further your knowledge.

In GNM, the concept of *disease* takes on an entirely different meaning, and the idea of a medicinal *cure*, a concoction that returns a patient to health, is rendered meaningless. A *disease* is most often the healing phase of your body's reaction to a psychic conflict shock. By the time you experience symptoms, by the time you notice something is wrong, your body is already healing, that is, reversing the actions it took in responding to the shock. Administering medicines at this time can interfere with the body's healing process, although certain medicines at certain times, may be warranted, may be helpful. In this view of disease, any *cure* can at best relieve a symptom, easing a patient's transition to

Definitions

health. At worst, it can interfere with the natural healing process, slowing recovery, and potentially cause new health insults.

GNM introduces many new concepts. I will be referring to them more than often, and group them here for convenience. This list is also recreated on my companion website: acriticallookat.com. If some of the abbreviations seem odd, it is because they derive from German, or Latin, where the words naturally differ from English.

- **DHS (Dirk Hamer syndrome).** A very difficult, highly acute, dramatic and isolating conflict shock, named after Dr. Hamer's son. According to GNM, all health insults of category F (cancer, diabetes, etc.) begin with a DHS. Think of a DHS as a figurative 2X4 upside your head that you didn't see coming.
- **SBS (significant biological special program).** The 2-phase coordinated myriad of processes your psyche, brain, and body undertake in response to a DHS. The second phase of an SBS is what many other medical modalities call disease. According to GNM, this program is never malignant or meaningless, but always serves a purpose, one that is biologically beneficial to the organism in times of emotional distress.
- **HH (Hamerschen herd).** Concentric ring patterns present on CT scans indicating the presence of an SBS. Dismissed as artifacts by mainstream medicine.
- **ST (sympathicotonia).** Normal day-time rhythm. The person is alert.
- **VT (vagotonia).** Normal night-time rhythm. The person is resting.
- **CA (conflict-active phase).** The first phase of an SBS. As the body is desperately trying to resolve a conflict, this phase is rarely marked by pain (dependent on the SBS), as pain is generally counterproductive to resolving the conflict.

- **CL (conflicto lysis).** Conflict resolution triggers the end of the first phase of an SBS, but only if the conflict is resolved.
- **PCL (post CL).** The second or healing phase of an SBS, when usually the distressing symptoms of what others call disease occur. It has three parts identified immediately below.
- **PCL-A.** First phase of healing. Marked by exudation (fluid buildup & swelling) and fever.
- **EC (epileptoid crisis).** A brief return to ST during which constriction expels the medium of healing (fluid). EC occurs between PCL-A and PCL-B.
- **PCL-B.** Second phase of healing. Marked by scarring and often pain.

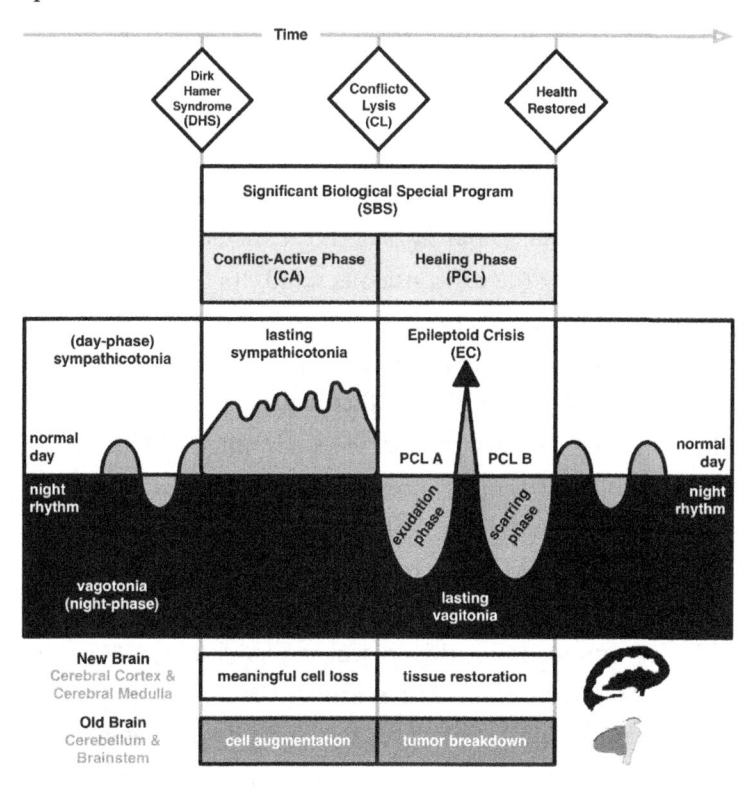

Progression of an SBS (read left to right, not top to bottom)

Definitions

> **First Biological Law (Iron Rule of Cancer)**[37]
> A DHS will trigger an SBS, producing an HH in a precise location of the brain as well as its corresponding organ.
>
> **Second Biological Law (The Law of 2 Phases)**
> Assuming a resolution to the conflict, an SBS will run in 2 phases, CA and PCL.
>
> **Third Biological Law**
> HH location in the brain and SBS phase determine cell loss/gain.
>
> **Fourth Biological Law**
> Microbes are not the cause of disease. They are directed by the brain to play a vital repair role in the SBS.
>
> **Fifth Biological Law**
> Every SBS (including any associated disease) is intended by Nature to help a being cope with unexpected distress.

The core tenet of GNM is the SBS. It is a reaction apparently intended to help ensure the survival of the individual. It is triggered by a DHS, which in effect, paralyzes the conscious mind, thereby necessitating action by the subconscious mind. Its goal is to (most often temporarily) modify biological capability to aid in overcoming a crisis. We are generally not aware that this is happening. This modification has a price, extracted if and after the conflict has been resolved. This price is generally referred to as disease, as the body must either rid itself of excess cells or rebuild cells it ulcerated in the conflict-active phase to return to a normal state. This 2-phase understanding of the nature of disease is unique to GNM in the medical paradigms I have studied.

Dr. Hamer summed up this discovery as follows: "All so-called diseases have a special biological meaning. While we used to regard Mother Nature as fallible and had the audacity to believe that She constantly made mistakes and caused breakdowns (malignant, senseless, degenerative cancerous growths, etc.) we can now see, as the scales fall from our eyes, that it was our ignorance and pride that were and are the only foolishness in our cosmos. Blinded, we brought upon ourselves this senseless, soulless and brutal medicine. Full of wonder, we can now understand for the first time that Nature is orderly (we already knew that), and every occurrence in Nature is meaningful, even in the framework of the whole, and that the events we called diseases are not senseless disturbances to be repaired by aspiring sorcerers. Nothing in Nature is meaningless, malignant or diseased."

Dr. Ryke Geerd Hamer was an internist at a cancer clinic in Germany. In 1978, his son Dirk was shot, eventually succumbing to his wounds. Shortly after Dirk's death, Dr. Hamer was diagnosed with testicular cancer.[38] After undergoing conventional treatment and recovering, Dr. Hamer wondered if his cancer was related somehow to Dirk's death. Having access to many cancer patients, he began talking to them to determine the circumstances leading up to their illness. All of them had experienced what Dr. Hamer realized was a psychic shock, that is, an unexpected event that rattled them, catching them totally off-guard, on the wrong foot, something they internalized, shared with nobody, and were unable to quickly resolve (thus, unknowingly triggering the involvement of their subconscious). Later Dr. Hamer named this conflict shock Dirk Hamer syndrome (DHS) in honor of his son. Analyzing Dr. Hamer's illness, the testicles produce sperm and hormones, such as testosterone, which affect both libido and virility. An increase in both would increase the chances of fathering another child to replace the loss. Per GNM, the result of such a cancer is precisely this increase.

How a potential DHS event is perceived is subjective. Different people may, and probably will, experience similar events differently. A devoutly religious person may chalk up a tragedy to God's will, and be sad, but not shocked, trusting in, and not questioning, God. A secular person may be devastated by the event and withdraw into himself,

Definitions

which, if perceived as a DHS, will, in turn, trigger an SBS to aid them in recovering from the tragedy. A baby or child will subjectively experience events differently than they would as an adult. Not being able to reach a binky could very well be shocking to an infant, whereas 20 years later, that same event would hopefully not even register.

The 1970s saw the introduction of CT scans, but by the 1980s, when Dr. Hamer was making his early discoveries of what was to become GNM, scans were still not commonplace. His first clue that the brain and organs were related to shock was when he noticed, in the CT scan of a heart patient, fluid on the heart rhythm center of the right side of the brain. Subsequent studies of more CT scans revealed concentric ring patterns, like a pebble makes when thrown into a pond. X-ray technicians dismissed these rings as artifacts, glitches in the system. CT scanners may very well produce ring artifacts. Does that mean that every ring pattern on a CT scan is an artifact? The manufacturer has certified that is not so.[39] Let's examine the evidence.

Dr. Hamer noticed that the concentric ring locations were not random; they were curiously only ever present in the parts of the brain thought to control the afflicted parts of his patient's bodies. In other words, the rings were centered on specific brain relays. This pairing was observed on many CT scans. Scans of a single patient from different angles produced the same ring patterns in identical brain locations. The chance that these are all artifacts is astronomically small. In GNM, these ring patterns are called Hamerschen Herd (HH). They indicate the presence of an SBS. They are a visual clue that a DHS has occurred.

Dr. Hamer systematically mapped HHs to afflicted organs, and further, to precise cellular structures within the body. Over time, he slowly produced an accurate map of the brain, linking the controlling brain area to the corresponding body part. He also noticed that as an

The Maverick Solution

SBS progressed from the active phase to the healing phase, the appearance of the HH changed, providing unexpected visual clues as to the state of the illness.

An essential concept in GNM is laterality or handedness[40]. Your dominant hand, determined by a simple clapping test (when clapping your hands, which hand is naturally on top?), is critical to realizing how a DHS is processed. It is an established fact that the right side of the brain controls the movement the left side of the body, and vice versa. Dr. Hamer observed that where an HH occurs is often dependent on laterality.[41] A DHS will effect a right-hander differently than a left-hander. In DHSs where laterality applies, a right-handed person will be affected on the left side of their body by conflicts with children or mother. Conflicts with everyone else, given a DHS, will impact the right side of their body. A left-hander will experience a mirror image of that scenario, child or mother on the right, everyone else on the left.

GNM proposes that an SBS is a biological response to threat. It is theorized that Homo Sapiens are an evolutionarily recent addition to life on earth. We are, as far as we can tell, the only life form capable of abstract thought. As an example of abstraction, we say that something stinks even though there is often nothing concrete to offend your nose. When we say we can't stomach something, it doesn't necessarily mean we have swallowed rotten food. We are capable of many such abstractions. GNM contends that both concrete and abstract events can be perceived as a DHS. It asserts that the brain does not distinguish between the two. This treating abstract like concrete is similar to dreams mimicking waking reality.

Microbes play a cleanup role during the healing phase of an SBS according to GNM. In fact, it is the Fourth Biological Law of GNM. In a previous chapter, titled *The Somatid,* I suggested that the pleomorphic

Definitions

nature of somatids could explain the sudden presence of microbes at healing sites throughout the body. Temperature changes in the body (fever), presumably directed by the brain, are implicated in the shape-shifting observed by Drs. Naessens and Béchamp. This pleomorphism occurs in not just humans, but all life, animal, and vegetable. Relatively little research has been done in this fascinating area. Questions such as *Exactly which microbes are unique to humans? Do all germs we associate with human illness spring from human somatids? Can a somatid from another species morph in the human body and impair human health?* and, *If so, is the mechanism of that illness basically a toxin response to its (foreign morphed somatid) waste products?* just begin to scratch the surface.

Your brain is continuously registering your environment, subconsciously noting all of your sensory input. When a DHS occurs, your brain associates much of those stimuli with the shock event, so that it can warn you should you again find yourself in a similar situation. Any sensory input: visual, audio, touch, taste, smell, emotion, can be linked to a DHS. GNM refers to these mental snapshots as tracks. When a track is encountered after the DHS has been resolved and normal health has resumed, the exposure may trigger the symptoms of the SBS associated with it, presumably to induce you to leave that environment. GNM might explain a rash for no apparent reason as having encountered a sensory input that essentially reminded your subconscious of a previous separation conflict (epidermis related health issues are viewed as separation conflicts in GNM). The rash would be your body's attempt to warn you of a potential separation shock. This understanding is central to GNM's explanation of chronic illness and allergies.

GNM professionals help you understand exactly why your body is not well, how it got that way, and what could return your health. Ideally, conflict resolution would follow quickly on the heels of a DHS thereby setting the stage for a natural quick recovery. All too frequently though,

The Maverick Solution

either the conflict is not resolved, or the healing is interrupted by tracks (which in effect simulate a DHS) or an actual DHS recurrence, leading to the often severe symptoms we call disease. If these snags in the SBS cycle are unintentional, that is, the product of ignorance, then the role of the GNM practitioner becomes clear. As educator and counselor, they seek to guide the patient through the SBS and back to health. Addressing symptoms may be appropriate, and referrals to specialists in other medical modalities may therefore be advised. GNM practitioners understand that Nature created the situation, and only Nature can reverse it, but along the way, symptom relief may be warranted. They avoid interfering with Nature's path and assist only where prudent. Always they seek to eliminate panic, which they know only exacerbates the problem, and may even lead to new health issues.

Let us unfold a typical illness scenario. You feel healthy and go about your day. You begin to notice that something is not right, health-wise. You may consume a tonic, and retire early. In the morning, you awake to find that you are not better, but worse. If you deem it necessary, you will visit a doctor for help. Typically, this doctor is one supported (paid) by health insurance plans; in the West, this is mostly allopathic. Your doctor will either help or not, depending on the illness. Either way, your doctor will be reacting to symptoms, making an educated guess, and proceeding with treatment. Any failure to help is generally not due to willingness, but rather, to ability, which is a function of your doctor's tools (knowledge, medicines, machines, procedures, etc.). If your doctor cannot help you, you may turn to alternative medicine. Again, this doctor is most probably reacting to symptoms, and again, will either help or not, with the same caveats. This cycle may repeat.

What if, you could know, ahead of time, that you might *fall ill*? What if, instead of reacting to symptoms, attacking those, and hoping that does the trick, you understand what the symptoms indicate, and where

Definitions

you are in this *disease* process? What if you knew what to expect? What if this knowledge alone was enough to ward off, or at least mitigate your illness? What if this knowledge enabled you to predict when your health would return, alleviating a large source of anxiety? What if this knowledge made the elimination of the chronic part of disease possible, allowing your health to return relatively quickly rather than to linger in illness year after year? What if your doctor shared this knowledge, and was able to guide you through any rough spots back to health? What if your doctor were expert at reading brain scans and was able to use them to confirm your illness suspicions and track your progress back to health? What if you both knew that Nature was doing her best to keep you alive, and that your symptoms were merely indicative of your body's return to health? Do you envision that scenario costing more or less than the mainstream approach of today? Do you envision that scenario being more or less effective and successful (in returning you to health) than the mainstream approach of today? Wouldn't you at least want such an option to be available for you to explore?

Well, it is, thanks to Dr. Hamer and a few students (see Reference section), turned teachers, who, recognizing the profound potential of this discovery, have helped to spread this knowledge. It requires your participation (you will play an active role in your recovery), your willingness to learn (ideally before any illness), and your confidence to trust your gut should this chapter ring true for you. I recommend you seek out the highest qualified practitioner you can find (visit their website, watch their videos, interview them, etc.), and start with a relatively innocuous illness, if you can. This process is no different than finding a trusted M.D., or N.D., or D.D.S. If you can nip a common cold in the bud using these methods, move up, try acne, athlete's foot, warts, etc. If you can conquer those, you should have a pretty good understanding of whether or not GNM works for you. It may seem strange to be so subjective about a health protocol, but if GNM is correct, remember that a DHS, which is where it all starts, is itself subjective, a personal reaction to events in your life.

GNM provides a framework based on 2-phase cell augmentation and ulceration that offers a compelling explanation as to how issues with your epidermis, your organ of touch, of feel, involve wanting to feel less. How issues with your dermis, your sub-skin so to speak, involve needing more physical protection. How issues with your nose, your organ of smell, involve wanting to smell less or smell more. How issues with your eyes, your organ of sight, involve wanting to see less. How issues with your ears, your organ of hearing, involve wanting to hear less. How issues with your brain, your organ of memory, among other things, sometimes involve wanting to remember less. How issues with your bladder, the organ used in the animal kingdom to mark territory, involve frustrations with territorial boundaries and are often family or work-related. How issues with the organs of digestion involve not being able to stomach something. How issues with bones and cartilage involve the desire for more physical prowess. Every part of the body has a purpose, and Nature may try to wring more performance from it from time to time in response to crisis. The return to normal health, or phase 2 of this process, often results in the symptoms that other medical paradigms call disease.

GNM proposes that surprise, surprise, the tissues compromised by illness are reacting to conflicts involving the core functionality of those tissues, in direct proportion to the intensity and duration of the conflict. It asserts that they have not been randomly attacked, except perhaps with toxins (see *The Problem* chapter). It proposes that Nature does not fail. It shows how microbes are directed by the organism to aid in healing, not to cause disease. It asserts that symptoms are clues to the underlying cause of illness, but that merely suppressing them will not assure your return to health. Finally, it demands that we understand

Definitions

that Nature is doing everything she can to ensure your survival, regardless of how consciously ignorant you are to her methods.

Embryology is the study of the development of embryos. A fertilized egg divides into a cluster called a blastocyst, which contains some cell differentiation. Around the two week mark, the blastocyst divides into three embryonic germ layers – endoderm, mesoderm, and ectoderm. All organs and tissues develop from these three layers. This pattern is not just a human phenomenon, as all animals share this process.

The next part of this explanation will benefit from a metonym of sorts. Embryology shows quite clearly that the embryos of most animals look very much alike early in their development. They all seem to share a similar core that becomes species distinct as it grows. Just how and why this happens is not the subject of this book, but I will refer to this metonym as evolution for brevity's sake. Some of you may disagree with current theories of evolution being responsible for the different species of our world. Again, this is not my subject, nor point, and I need a handy word to express compartmentalization – I choose evolution as this word.

From an evolutionary standpoint, the oldest part of the brain is the brainstem. This part of the brain controls organs that derive from the endoderm. These organs are responsible for consuming and eliminating. Think of their target as a morsel. A *food morsel* is handled by the esophagus, stomach, and intestines, an *air morsel* by the lung alveoli, a *sound morsel* by the Eustachian tubes and middle ear, a *water morsel* by the kidney collecting tubules, a *visual morsel* by the tear glands. DHSs affecting the brainstem are all morsel conflicts. During the conflict-active (CA) phase, there is cell proliferation, with a reversal, or tuberculosis aided cell breakdown during the PCL (healing) phase. Tissues controlled by the brainstem include kidney collecting tubules, small intestine, duodenum, pancreas, liver, nucleus of acoustic nerve, pharynx, uterus mucosa, fallopian tubes, prostate gland, esophagus (lower third), lung alveoli, stomach, sigmoid colon, rectum and bladder mucosa, and the glandular foreskin of the penis.

The next oldest part is the midbrain, which is actually an area of the brainstem. It controls organs that derive from the endoderm; smooth musculature throughout the body. It is responsible for peristalsis or moving the morsel through the body. DHSs involving the midbrain are all conflicts of insufficient peristalsis. During the CA phase, there is cell proliferation (a local increase of smooth muscle tissue), with colic, but no cell removal during the PCL phase. Tissues controlled by the midbrain include the smooth musculature of the ingoing and outgoing intestine, uterus, heart muscle, and blood vessels.

Continuing evolutionarily, the next oldest part of the brain is the cerebellum. It controls organs derived from mesodermal tissue and is responsible for protection. DHSs involving the cerebellum are all attack conflicts, either physical or perceived (e.g. attacks on one's integrity). During the CA phase (SBS phase 1), there is cell proliferation, with a reversal, or tuberculosis aided cell breakdown during the PCL phase (SBS phase 2). Tissues controlled by the cerebellum include breast glands, pleura and peritoneum, pericardium, and corium skin.

These first three sections of the brain are collectively known as the old-brain. The final two sections, explored below, are known as the new-brain.

The cerebral medulla evolved next, and is responsible for our structure (bones, cartilage, etc.). It also controls organs that derive from the mesoderm. DHSs involving the cerebral medulla are all self-devaluation conflicts, where we experience a conflict shock due to not

Definitions

being able to perform physically as before, or as we would like, or expect. During the CA phase, there is cell necrosis (tissue loss), with a reversal, or cell restoration (resulting in more tissue than before) during the PCL phase. Tissues controlled by the cerebral medulla include striated part of myocardium, arms, legs, shoulders, cervical, thoracic and lumbar vertebrae, adrenal cortex, pelvis, spleen, knees, feet, testicles and ovaries, and kidney parenchyma.

The youngest part of the brain, the cerebral cortex, controls all the rest: organs deriving from the ectoderm. Territorial and separation conflicts affect these parts of the body. These conflicts are marked by either tissue loss during the CA phase, followed by cell restoration during the PCL phase, or by functional impairment during CA, followed by renormalization of function during PCL.

The biological advantage of SBSs occurs during the first phase (CA) with the exception being those controlled by the cerebral medulla, in which it appears at the end of the second phase (PCL-B).

Thomas Jefferson observed, "If a nation expects to be ignorant and free, in a state of civilization, it expects what never was and never will be." Jefferson viewed liberty as a gift from God. Keeping it requires an understanding of what it is, and subsequently, why it is important. Casting the quote in a GNM light, it reads, "If you expect to be ignorant and healthy, in a state of civilization, with all of its potential conflicts, you expect what never was and never will be." Most people view health as a gift from God (or Nature, if you prefer). I submit that maintaining it requires an understanding of how it is sometimes lost. The good news here is that GNM does not demand the comprehension of a medical professional. A layman's curiosity and understanding will suffice, augmented of course by professional expertise in dealing with actual health concerns.

The Medicine

Medicine is the chemical (or energy in the case of Homeopathy) component of a *cure* as discussed previously. Patents protect some, while others are naturally occurring compounds.

In the patent pharmaceutical space, after centuries of seemingly random chance discoveries, trial and error methods are giving way to designed drugs.[42] The old techniques resulted in a failure rate of 95%, making the drugs that did make their way into circulation very expensive, as profits on these 5% had to pay for the failures as well. The trial and error method, of course, reveals nothing of cause, forcing their proponents to admit ignorance as to the reason those drugs actually worked.[43] With designed drugs, molecular simulations enable researchers to create medicines specifically designed to have a particular molecular effect. The closer the simulation mimics reality, the better the results of this method. A potential fly in this ointment is that such realism indirectly assumes precise knowledge of the cause of illnesses, a proposition in the allopathic world that is unfortunately laid waste to in the chapters to come. At present, the hope is a reduction in failure rate from 95% to 67%, making less expensive pharmaceuticals possible.

In the herbal or alternative space, remedies are discovered by accident, by trial and error, by observing animal instinct, and by shamanic insight usually under psychotropic influence. Compiled and corrected over millennia, this record is extensive and of proven practical

Definitions

value. Cause is however, largely a mystery; that it works is far better understood than how it works.

Looking at how medicines work through the lens of GNM,[44] we can see that the Second Biological Law (the law of 2 phases), governs the response to a drug. Patented or natural makes no difference in this observation. This law asserts that when your normal day/night rhythm is interrupted by a conflict shock (DHS), you will maintain a state of high alert (ST) until the conflict is resolved. After which you will transition into an opposite, or rest state (VT) until your brain has reversed the actions it undertook during the conflict-active (CA) phase. The two phases will be equal in duration, barring relapses or tracks. The brain maintains these states chemically through the use of stress hormones, either by releasing more (in ST), or less (in VT), from a baseline level.

Remember that this state switch hinges on the resolution of the conflict that started it all. It is almost always biologically advantageous to resolve conflicts as soon as possible. Higher levels of stress hormones make it difficult to sleep,[45] so that your brain can spend longer periods of time resolving the conflict. They also prepare the entire body for *fight or flight*, helpful should the conflict resolution require physical exertion. Once the conflict is resolved, the body lowers the stress hormone level, inducing rest and sleep, and instigates repairs, which often result in the symptoms we call disease.

Drugs directly or indirectly modify this hormone state, acting as either a stimulant or a sedative, increasing or decreasing stress. Most of our *disease* symptoms occur after conflict resolution, when the body is in VT. Common remedies for diseases in this state are stimulants, which induce stress, countering the symptoms of the healing phase. GNM views drugs that are claimed to boost the immune system as stimulants.

The Medicine

They effectively prolong the healing phase by reducing the intensity of healing symptoms (echinacea, vitamin C, caffeine, etc.) Some symptoms will occur during the ST phase when the body has raised its stress level through hormones. A typical desire in a high-stress state is to lower the stress through sedatives. This has the effect of dulling focus on a resolution to the conflict, prolonging the conflict-active phase as well.

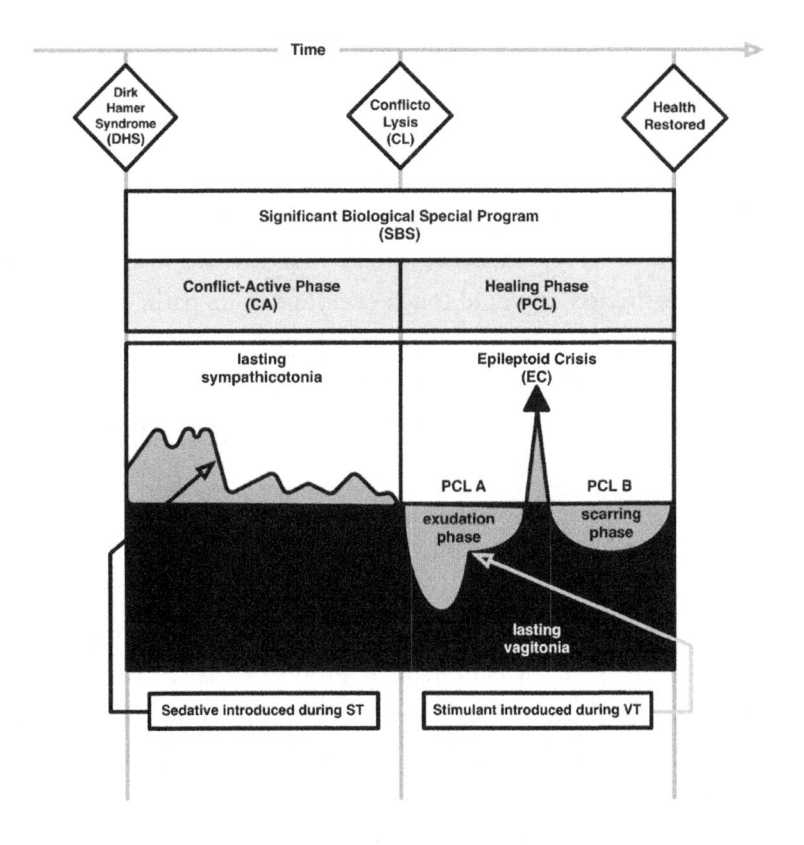

```
                                Time
         ◇                         ◇                         ◇
      Dirk                      Conflicto                   Health
      Hamer                      Lysis                     Restored
    Syndrome                      (CL)
      (DHS)

    ┌─────────────────────────────────────────────────────┐
    │          Significant Biological Special Program      │
    │                        (SBS)                         │
    ├──────────────────────────┬──────────────────────────┤
    │   Conflict-Active Phase  │      Healing Phase       │
    │           (CA)           │          (PCL)           │
    ├──────────────────────────┼──────────────────────────┤
    │         lasting          │    Epileptoid Crisis     │
    │      sympathicotonia     │          (EC)            │
    │                          │                          │
    │                          │  PCL A         PCL B     │
    │                          │                          │
    │                          │ exudation    scarring    │
    │                          │   phase       phase      │
    │                          │                          │
    │                          │        lasting           │
    │                          │       vagitonia          │
    └──────────────────────────┴──────────────────────────┘
    │  Sedative introduced during ST │ Stimulant introduced during VT │
```

In this view, stimulants given during an active (CA & EC) phase will exacerbate the stress symptoms; if you have trouble sleeping, would you drink coffee (a stimulant)? Sedatives taken during a healing phase (PCL A & B) will do likewise to the healing symptoms; would you down shots of alcohol (a sedative) with a stopped up head from a bad cold?

The Epidemic

There is a phenomenon wherein many people in a geographic area fall ill at roughly the same time; epidemics are a familiar health topic. That they occur is a fact. There are several theories as to why they occur.

An early now disregarded theory was that bad, or night air, arriving from rotting material could cause illness. Naturally, since airflow is generally not restricted, it would touch everyone in its path, creating the requirements for an epidemic. The term given this foul air was miasma.[46] Proponents viewed epidemics as mass poisonings. It was a forerunner to the Germ Theory of disease (and epidemics), giving way to this new idea around 1880.

Louis Pasteur successfully championed the Germ Theory[47] of disease. Versions of this theory had been bandied about for centuries. It replaced the *bad air* of the Miasma Theory with germs, becoming a core principle of the mainstream medical paradigm. It proposes that disease-causing microorganisms (pathogens) are external to the body invading us through the air we breathe, the food we eat, the water we drink or the substances we touch. Thus, Germ Theory can be seen as a refinement of the Miasma Theory by isolating the active ingredient in bad air that is implicated in causing the disease. It then also expands on the Miasma Theory by including other vectors for these pathogens other than just air.

The Epidemic

Traditional Chinese Medicine (TCM) also regards epidemics as an external attack via heaven (airborne) or earth (direct contact), albeit traditionally not from a pathogen source, as the theories were born in the 16th century, long before Germ Theory. Warm disease[48] (Wen Bing) and hot disease (Re Bing) initially affect the exterior of the patient before proceeding to the interior.

Ayurveda seems to take a similar approach as TCM, and I was unable to ascertain their understanding of how transmission of the disease occurs from one person to the next, only that it does.

Naturopathy generally favors the Terrain Theory of disease over the Germ Theory, stressing a clean body as the best defense against illness. From this, I gather that an epidemic would indicate a significant population would all have to have compromised terrains. Just how they would all simultaneously take ill is not well explained in this view other than perhaps toxins.

German New Medicine explains that disease is the result of a reaction to psychic shock. That shock may be personal, or it may be communal, that is, affecting a community instead of just a single individual. When a community experiences a shock, then it is logical to expect that more than one person will be affected.

GNM explains the lung tuberculosis epidemic (Spanish Flu) after World War 1[49] as a mass conflict resolution (end of the war) of a territorial-worry conflict, which affects the bronchial mucosa. This epidemic may also have been exacerbated by mass accidental overdosing of a soon to be very popular pain medication that was just introduced into the global market.[50]

Definitions

It also similarly explains measles epidemics, although the conflict is different, and not nearly as traumatic as war. Measles is a disease of the skin. GNM equates skin diseases with separation conflicts. Young children are more apt to be shocked by that first big separation from their family and as such, more prone to measles. Since school begins for all at the same time, the conditions are ripe for a communal DHS. After a short period, when the young students realize that their new teacher is not some monster, and is probably quite pleasant, and there are many fun things to do and new friends to be found, a resolution to the conflict ensues. Those affected are likely to manifest symptoms (healing phase) at roughly the same time, triggering a measles epidemic panic.

Nature employs this mechanism in all animals, not just humans. Imagine what kinds of DHS events are experienced by domestic animals in factory farms where the conditions are, shall we say, less than ideal for the livestock. Since they are all exposed to the same conditions, how likely is it that a majority will suffer simultaneous shocks? Does that scenario offer a rational explanation for avian and swine flu scares (poultry and pork factory farms)?[51]

The bubonic plague that ravaged Europe in the Middle Ages is credited with killing roughly half of that population and is a poster child for epidemics. Popular culture places the cause as a dreaded skin disease, though it has recently been argued[52] that the real culprit in the Black Death was pneumonic plague, which afflicts the lungs. GNM relates such a (lung) condition with a death-fight (air morsel) conflict, one of not being able to breathe (not being able to consume enough air morsels). The black boils that give the disease its name are rooted in the corium skin, indicating an attack conflict. Remember that in the Middle Ages, Pasteur's germ theory had yet to be imagined, and people envisioned the cause of the plague to be God's will.[53] It is easy to conflate a death panic with being unable to flee God's wrath, and simultaneously to see how the plague spread so quickly, given the God-fearing nature of the public at the time. These are merely two different ways of explaining the same facts.

The modern epidemic of AIDS has claimed 35 million lives since the mid-1980s, with an equal number still living with the affliction. AIDS is a collection of symptoms in search of a disease. Mainstream medicine envisions a virus as culprit, the dreaded human immunodeficiency virus (HIV). This despite the fact that some who test positive for HIV[54] show no symptoms of AIDS, and likewise, some who show symptoms of AIDS, test negative for HIV, obliterating all four of Koch's Postulates.

What does GNM have to say about AIDS? Well, the collection of diseases that reside under the AIDS umbrella[55] each have their distinct causes. Each is individual. Together, all at once, they define AIDS, and it is easy to see how, manifesting simultaneously, they can overwhelm a person. An obvious question at this point is, why would a person experience all of these diseases at once? Kaposi sarcomas are melanomas. They form on the corium skin in response to an attack conflict. The first victims of AIDS were homosexual men in an age where many gays were still *in the closet*. How many felt attacked for their sexuality? The biological conflict associated with the lymph nodes is a self-devaluation conflict. For me, it is easy to imagine that the pressure to hide a fundamental part of oneself, could result in intense feelings of self-devaluation. Prolonged swelling of the lymph happens to be another symptom of AIDS. Yet another is sores of the mouth, anus, or genitals. The epidermis reacts to separation conflicts, with sores presenting during the healing phase at the point(s) of conflict. The conflict can be one of wanting to separate, or not wanting to. Seen in the light of the highly promiscuous gay scene of the 1980s, coupled with the social stigma of homosexuality at the time, it is not difficult to imagine either conflict. Pneumonia is another symptom of AIDS and is viewed by GNM

Definitions

as bronchitis (territorial-fear conflict: bullying, frightening medical diagnosis, etc.) coupled with an abandonment or existence (self-devaluation} conflict, resulting in kidney collecting tubule syndrome. Again, for me, it is not difficult to imagine how homosexuals could be affected by all of these conflicts, leading to a diagnosis of AIDS.

Dr. Hamer had this to say about AIDS (HIV) testing:[56] "If a patient suffers a DHS with a territorial conflict that entails a smegma track, e.g., a man has 'smelled' his rival's smegma when catching his partner 'red handed', his AIDS test will be positive. AIDS is not a disease. It is merely a harmless allergy test, which has intentionally and falsely been labeled a disease." Note that he was not saying that the many diseases under the AIDS umbrella were harmless. He was criticizing the AIDS (HIV) test and noting that AIDS, by itself, is not a disease, but a group of symptoms, which is the very definition of the word *syndrome* (see chapter *Liver and Gallbladder:Mainstream* for an in-depth discussion of viral testing).

Ebola is a modern-day scare that threatens to reach epidemic status in parts of West Central Africa, though the number of victims pales to say, victims of influenza. Mainstream medical sources report a death rate of 50% for those afflicted. Symptoms apparently include fever, severe headache, muscle pain, weakness, fatigue, diarrhea, vomiting, stomach pain, and unexplained hemorrhage. That people show these signs and die (quickly) is unquestioned, at least by me. Why they do, is again, theory. Mainstream medicine blames a virus. Maybe, but it appears there are serious questions about the reliability of the diagnostic test,[57] and the symptoms could also easily be interpreted as poisoning. Just such a report involving formaldehyde in compromised Liberian water wells leading to ebola symptoms[58] is understandably met with skepticism, due in no small part to the energy-based geopolitical instability of the region. Why then is the virus theory not subject to the same scrutiny?

The Placebo

Doctors who administer medicine (patent or natural) to their patients have observed for centuries, that often, all that is required of a drug, is that the patient believes in its effectiveness. In randomized control trials (RCT), inert pills that mimic active pills in appearance and taste are used as a control to judge the effective function of a given medicine. The assumptions are that test subject will not know if they are taking a medicine or not and that the placebo pill will have no effect. Now remind me, what did your mother tell you about assuming?

Turns out, even when they work, up to 50% of a drug's impact may be due to the placebo effect.[59] A logical assumption is that the patient expects the drug to help, or put another way, their brain does. To me, that's a pretty big clue in unraveling the mystery of health. The mind is intricately linked to health somehow.

The big question then is how? How does the brain take the information that help is on its way to morph illness to health? Of the five solutions outlined previously (Mainstream, Ancient, Royal, Alternative and Maverick), which, if any of them, account for this observed behavior? That placebos work is a fact; how they work is a theory. You decide which strikes closest to the mark. You decide which theory explains this phenomenon best.

The five solutions can be roughly broken into three categories. The first is highly technical and seemingly focused on sophisticated

Definitions

diagnostic tools, and on patented symptom suppression strategies, i.e. on disease management. It is firmly rooted in the Germ Theory of disease. It contains only the Mainstream solution.

The second category seeks to mainly assist the body in returning the patient to health, relying heavily on remedies found in Nature, and cataloged over millennia. It also generally reacts to symptoms, albeit with a seemingly more gentle touch. It uses energy theories (vital force), skeletal alignment strategies, the Germ Theory as well as the Terrain Theory of disease in seeking solutions to illness. It is generally holistic in practice. This diverse group contains the Ancient, Royal and Alternative Solutions.

The third category offers precise explanations as to the cause of diseases, relying on the diagnostic and, for medical emergencies only, the surgical techniques of the first category and traditional symptom relief remedies from the second, and if necessary first, categories. This category finally and fully explains the Terrain Theory of disease, and soundly rejects the Germ Theory. It contains only the Maverick solution.

As I feature specific health conditions in the section ahead, I will illustrate my understanding of how the first and third (and occasionally second) categories view each ailment. In other words, I will explore their theories, while interjecting my opinions thereof. This will be followed by my audit of the current state of professional care for the condition. The second category, in my opinion, is unfortunately too broad to do anything other than generalize about conditions. For this reason it is necessarily underrepresented in the next section. This broad brush approach yields an admittedly vague general understanding along the lines of use: herbs, massage, skeletal manipulation, acupuncture and diet and lifestyle changes to attempt to normalize balance and harmony in an effort to return a patient to health. While this is a gross oversimplification of sophisticated medical modalities, it is by my understanding, essentially correct.

I will take the opportunity before getting into various examples of category F health issues (cancer, diabetes, heart disease, etc.) to reiterate my earlier disclaimer. This book is **not** intended as a substitute for professional medical advice. I am **not** a doctor, and therefore you must not rely on this material for medical treatment. If you have any specific health concerns, you would be wise to consult a qualified health professional. The chapters that follow in the next section are intended to illuminate my understanding (from research and first and second hand knowledge) of existing medical practices, and should only be viewed as informative, never diagnostic.

Initial disease definitions at the beginning of each chapter in the next section reflect common usage. Throughout this section, I highlight groups that have organized to focus on a particular disease or condition. I do this to give a sense of scope to their (mostly mainstream) efforts and to contrast that with the mainstream understanding of the causes of disease. All information I present about them was learned from their respective websites and is heavily referenced.

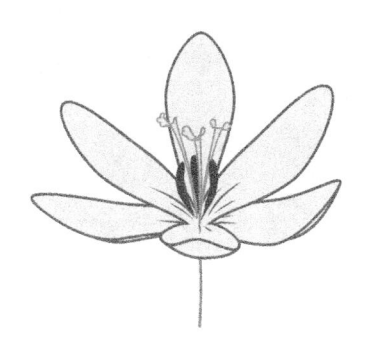

Healthcare

Allergies

An allergy is an immune system overreaction to a substance (allergen) it considers harmful. Antibodies called immunoglobulin E (IgE), responds to the allergen, producing the symptoms we refer to as allergy.

Allergies are not anywhere near the top of the list of most deadly diseases. I have given them their own chapter as they are a pivotal topic in GNM.

Organization

The leading patient organization for people with asthma and allergies was founded in 1953.[60] They have been using education, advocacy, and research in support of allergy and asthma patients for close to 65 years now. Their total revenues for 2015 were $3,963,720.[61]

The origins of another such organization[62] dates back to the 1920s, so they are fast approaching their century mark. In 2017, they reportedly awarded almost $1 million for allergy or immunology research projects.

The federal budget for Allergies (see *Appendix*) is low compared to other illnesses, but still, $85 million for 2017 is not a trivial sum.

Mainstream Theory

Allopathy theorizes that failures of the immune system in mistaking harmless substances as dangerous invaders, results in the inflammations commonly referred to as allergies.[63] This definition highlights a core allopathic axiom: that in otherwise healthy bodies, Nature makes mistakes and occasionally reacts needlessly. I could find no mention of why your body would make such blunders, or how needless reactions would benefit your existence or survival.

The standard therapy for allergies is immunotherapy, wherein a purified allergen is injected subcutaneously in increasing amounts over time in an effort to desensitize the patient to the allergen. Short of that, all manner of pharmaceuticals are offered to combat the numerous symptoms of allergies.

Conventional medicine sees the cause of allergies as a confused immune system, triggered by the allergen, in keeping with the general allopathic invader perspective. The reason for the confusion is blamed on either genetics or the environment. As the environment affects everyone, and not everyone has allergies, the argument logically reduces to genetics, which does nothing to explain why allergies seem to generationally ebb and flow. Peanut allergies were rare to nonexistent when I was young; now they are relatively epidemic. I'm not that old; peanut butter did exist when I was a kid, and it was well acquainted with my lunchbox. Could this spike have something to do with the introduction of the 1970s of a new peanut variety,[64] which dramatically increased the supply of this staple? I am not suggesting that this new peanut is directly responsible for peanut allergies. I am suggesting, in a market environment such as found in the USA, that spectacular increases in food yields tend to exert downward pressures on prices, resulting in higher (more widespread) consumption of that food. Did an increase in the consumption of peanut butter (any peanut butter) in the 1970s (continuing to the present) lead, however indirectly, to a rise in peanut allergies? I think it did; the question is how? If genes are implicated, why are they affected by a yummy and now less expensive and therefore ubiquitous food?

Allopathy counsels abstinence or avoidance as a front line of defense, as it is difficult to imagine how their usual arsenal of surgery and radiation would be of any help. Drugs to lessen symptoms are a secondary line of defense, in particular, epinephrine, as an emergency response to anaphylaxis, a potentially fatal reaction.

Alternative Theory

NAET, ([Dr. Devi] Nambudripad's allergy elimination techniques) blends selective energy balancing, testing and treatment procedures from acupuncture/acupressure, allopathy, chiropractic, nutritional therapies, and kinesiology. It defines allergy as a blockage of energy flow in the body, borrowing the Ancient solution's way of looking at the problem. Treatment requires total avoidance of the offending allergen for 25 hours. It boasts 12,000+ practitioners worldwide. NAET claims an 80-90% success rate for its protocol,[65] and has had at least some of that claim verified by independent researchers.[66]

Maverick Theory

As explained in the chapter *The Maverick Solution*, the brain, at the instant of a DHS (conflict shock), can associate sensory inputs at that moment with the conflict. Experienced again at a later time, these *tracks* can trigger the same symptoms that accompanied the SBS (2-phase reaction to DHS). They are warnings of a possible new shock but are only ever recognized as such if the person is familiar with GNM.

To understand how tracks and allergies are associated, we need to remember the second GNM law, the law of 2 phases. When we encounter a track, the psyche is immediately put back into a conflict-active (CA) state (SBS phase 1), but since the conflict has been resolved, the brain transitions quickly to the first healing phase (SBS phase 2), PCL-A, which is marked by inflammation and swelling. In other words, typical allergy symptoms. According to GNM, allergies can be eliminated by recognizing, becoming conscious of, the DHS associated with the track. Once made consciously aware, your subconscious will dissociate the two, and the allergen will no longer trigger that response.

The allergy symptoms are actually clues to what the associated DHS was. Hay fever (stuffy/runny nose) indicates the former DHS was a stink or scent conflict. A rash (hives, dermatitis, rosacea, etc.) indicates an earlier separation conflict. Diarrhea upon eating certain foods signifies a previous undigestible-morsel conflict. Difficulty breathing stems from a territorial-fear conflict. Although this is now changing, due to restrictions imposed because of the scope of the present-day allergy problem, peanut butter and jelly sandwiches were long a staple of school children's lunches (perhaps due in part to a drop in PB prices). School lunchtimes are often less supervised than classrooms and can force a mingling of children from differing age groups (unlike the classroom). Could this environment breed territorial conflicts, wherein the omnipresent PBJ sandwich with its distinctly delicious aroma is registered as a track?

Constant exposure to tracks in this fashion can result in a chronic condition, where the body doesn't finish healing but is repeatedly thrown back into a conflict-active (CA) state, followed immediately by the healing state. GNM refers to this as a hanging-healing, which may also be the result of a repeated DHS.

Audit

Mainstream medicine sees the cause of allergic reactions as Nature mistaking an otherwise harmless substance as an invader. Familiar symptoms such as watery eyes, sneezing, skin rashes, etc., are evidence of a battle waging between these allergens and your immune system. It is a continuance of the concept of the human battlefield, proposed by the Germ Theory of disease. Many alternative medical paradigms embrace the same explanation but differ in their treatment. GNM offers an end to these situations, as it has identified root cause and therefore a clear path to healing.

From an audit viewpoint, relatively little money is spent on these issues, as most are merely inconvenient. Still, $85 million annually (in the USA alone) is far too large a sum to simply waste, which is precisely what is happening if Dr. Hamer is correct in his assessment of allergies.

Allergies that cause anaphylactic reactions are often serious medical emergencies, demanding an immediate medical response. The mainstream solution is an injection of epinephrine (another word for adrenalin which constricts blood vessels), where current product pricing seems to be in an extreme state of flux,[67] ranging from almost free to north of $300 per dose. Unfortunately for the patient, this approach is another example of disease management, an often lifelong prognosis.

Bones And Cartilage

This chapter deals with disorders of bones and cartilage other than cancer (see *Cancer* chapter).

Arthritis is a painful inflammation and stiffness of the joints.

Osteoporosis is brittle bones.

Organizations

The preeminent charitable organization for arthritis[68] was founded in 1948. Their total revenues for 2015 were $81,122,060.[69] They have cataloged more than 100 different types of arthritis and related conditions in their nearly 70 year existence, but admit that the disease is not well understood. From this, we know that they have done a bang-up job of classifying the issue, of identifying medical problems collectively called arthritis. They can readily identify the symptoms, and can thus direct treatment, but have decidedly less understanding of why arthritis occurs, and so, in my opinion, little chance at present of finding a cure, which is their stated goal. This seems to be a common thread among health charities.

The leading osteoporosis charity was founded 33 years ago in 1984. It is the only health organization dedicated solely to osteoporosis and bone health in the United States. Their revenue for 2016 was $3,306,808.[70] They too, according to their website, seem to have a better

Healthcare

understanding of what osteoporosis is, than what causes it, although they do provide an extensive list of diseases, condition and medical procedures that may cause bone loss[71]. A prestigious medical research group[72] dispenses with all ambiguity and simply opines that bone mass loss overtakes bone mass creation in people in their early to mid 20s, in effect saying that bone loss will happen to everyone; it is merely a matter of degree (which at some point delineates osteoporosis).

Funding for arthritis research at the federal level (see *Appendix*) is even higher, averaging $230 million annually for the past five years. Federal funding for osteoporosis has hovered around the $150 million mark in that same period. Unsurprisingly, as with every government medical research program, most of the money is spent exploring mainstream theories of health.

The oldest and largest dental nonprofit in the USA was founded in 1859 and represents more than 161,000 member dentists. It differs from similar groups listed in this book who are actively seeking to rid the world of their particular disease, in that, from what I can surmise from their website, their goal is simply better dental health.[73] Perhaps nearly 160 years of research and battling the sweet tooth has tempered their outlook. Dental care is an enormous industry, with annual spending[74] projected to reach $185 billion in 2025, a 52% increase from the $122 billion spent in 2016.

Mainstream Theory

Mainstream medicine has shown that peak bone loss in women tends to coincide with menopause[75] and theorizes that estrogen plays a role in bone density. However, roughly half of all women 50 years or older do not suffer from low bone mass,[76] yet every woman experiences a similar reduction in estrogen. Furthermore, roughly 20% of all osteoporosis patients are men, who do not experience menopause. Clearly, it is not as simple as low estrogen = low bone mass, a common misconception. In fact, mainstream research points to a different cause of low bone mass in men, namely low testosterone.[77]

Calcium and vitamin D deficiencies are also suspect in osteoporosis. In the elderly, this can have many causes, but regardless of how the deficiencies occur, any nutrient issue falls under the heading of malnutrition, or as I labeled them in the chapter *The Problem*, category B, and therefore outside of the scope of this book.

Osteoporosis has been found in almost every bone in the human body, though bone mass testing is usually measured at the hip by a DEXA scan.[78] Not everyone though is affected in the same skeletal area: some have weakened hips, others are impacted in the spine, while still others suffer shoulder issues. Why?

Experts in the medical mainstream lament that arthritis is not well understood despite being common. Typical for allopathy, what happens (symptoms) is detailed. Why it happens (cause) is uncertain. Symptom management is therefore the current allopathic strategy for arthritis.

Teeth are a special form of bone that mainstream medicine has isolated medically. Dentistry handles problems with the teeth and is a discipline unto itself. Doctors of Medicine (MD) do not concern themselves with teeth, and Doctors of Dental Surgery (dentists) only concern themselves with teeth. This may have something to do with dentistry historically being associated with barbers, a decidedly non-medical profession. Regardless of the source of this schism, allopathic dentistry aligns with its MD counterparts by using its tools (drugs, surgery and radiation, this last for diagnosis, not treatment). Allopathic dentistry forces crooked teeth into alignment, removes and replaces decayed teeth, repairs compromised portions of teeth with artificial materials such as amalgam (50% mercury, the rest silver, tin, copper, and trace metals), ceramic composites and gold.

Few seem to ask why teeth are crooked. It is simply accepted as fact, and the symptoms are addressed by mechanical means (braces). The cause of tooth decay is postulated to be sugar-loving bacteria, so emphasis is placed on the cleaning of teeth and the avoidance of excessive sweets. Chemicals (fluoride compounds) and coatings are slathered on teeth to harden and seal them artificially. Despite all this, 90+% of the US population will experience tooth decay over their lifetime, with the average number of missing, decayed or filled teeth of those over 60 approaching 20.[79] What is more likely? Are most people ignoring dentist recommendations to preserve your teeth because they secretly enjoy the pain and expense of tooth decay, or are those recommendations perhaps missing a major culprit in oral health?

Adding fluoride to public water supplies as a method for hardening teeth is strongly recommended by dental authorities.[80] Used in this manner, the fluoride added to water is a drug,[81] and as such, is the only doctor recommended drug, of which I am aware, whose dose is seemingly irrelevant. Given a fluoridated public water supply, those who bathe often, or spend long hours in swimming pools are subject to larger doses of fluoride (absorption through skin) than those who don't.[82] A similar situation exists with drinking fluoridated tap water; as daily consumption varies widely. Lastly, the quantity of water, and therefore fluoride, used in food preparation is difficult to monitor. The total dose of fluoride a person receives is thus practically unknowable. The utility company knows how much fluoride they add to their water supply, but I fail to see how they can have any way of knowing just how much of it made its way into their consumers.

As with most drugs, fluoride carries a risk of side effects.[83] The benefit of any drug is typically weighed against its detriment to health. To administer a drug effectively, dose must be known. Even oxygen and water, our two most essential consumables, are toxic, to the point of being lethal, in high enough doses. In prescribing all other drugs of which I am aware, age and weight are relevant factors in determining dose. Apparently, fluoride stands alone in dismissing these requirements. The risk of our general consumption of fluoride is therefore impossible to ascertain with any certainty. Limiting fluoride to toothpaste would largely mitigate this problem, while simultaneously enabling those who view fluoride as toxic to opt out of consuming it. It is noteworthy that in 1997, the Food and Drug Administration (FDA) of the US federal government ordered all toothpaste manufacturers to add a warning to their fluoride toothpastes – "Keep out of reach of children under 6 years of age. If you accidentally swallow more than used for brushing, seek professional help or contact a poison control center immediately." A stern warning presumably meant for a significant risk.

The typical manufacturers recommended *dose* of toothpaste is pea-sized. The typical toothpaste advertisement routinely shows the entire top of the brush completely covered in paste, many times the recommendation. How much is fluoride is accidentally swallowed? How much is absorbed through the interior skin of the mouth? How much of *do not swallow* are little children expected to comprehend, especially when fluoridated toothpaste marketed to children is often flavored like candy?

Alternative Theory

Chiropractic is an alternative medical paradigm that focuses on joint misalignments as the cause of many human health issues. As such,

Healthcare

Doctors of Chiropractic have an excellent working knowledge of the skeletal framework. This specialty can treat the symptoms of osteoporosis but I believe that they share the same understanding of cause as the mainstream, one with many open questions.

Tourette syndrome has long been thought to be a neurological disorder by mainstream medicine. A large organization dedicated to this condition[84] describes it as a childhood-onset, neurodevelopment disorder, and believes the causes to be genetic and environmental. Taking a different approach, a dentist in Virginia, Dr. Brendan Stack,[85] noticed that his treatment of TMJ (with an oral device that realigned the jaw) relieved Tourette symptoms immediately. His theory is that facial nerves are being pinched by slipped or out of place, TMJ disks, resulting in the facial tics and vocal spasms of Tourette. The oral device, which creates a space between the upper and lower teeth (a custom fitted, functional equivalent of a stack of popsicle sticks), appears to relieve the pressure on said nerves, resulting in what appears to be instant relief. Microsurgery is available to set the TMJ disks back in their proper place permanently. The observation that the affliction is childhood-onset provides a perfect segue into the discoveries of my next guest.

In the first half of the 20th century, a dentist from Cleveland, Ohio set out to study isolated groups of humans. Dr. Weston Price[86] sought to rigorously document the connection between diet and oral health. His insightful recommendations concerning the proper preparation of grains (sprouting, fermentation, or natural leavening), and high caloric intake of animal fat have unfortunately found only the smallest of toeholds in the West despite a preponderance of anecdotal evidence showing the benefits of such a diet. The deleterious effects on oral health once these isolated groups adopted a modern diet heavy in processed foods is a matter of record. These adverse effects extended to the malformation of the oral cavity in children to the decay of teeth.[87] What is done for the convenience and profits of food producers is apparently not always best for the health of the consumer. Imagine that.

Maverick Theory

GNM relates issues with bone and cartilage to conflicts regarding a reduction in one's assessment of self-worth. These parts of the body provide the structural support of the whole. The stronger the conflict, the *deeper* the SBS (2-phase reaction to conflict-shock) will reach. Severe conflicts affect the bones, medium conflicts, cartilage and lymph, and slight conflicts can affect connective tissue and blood vessels.

This category of DHS (conflict shock) is a self-devaluation conflict. GNM proposes that when a person suffers such a conflict, their body will automatically attempt to make it stronger. It does this by deconstructing the area threatened by attack during the conflict-active (CA) period, preparing it for a more dense rebuild, which then occurs after the conflict is resolved, typically marked by the return of self-esteem. Biologically, the SBS is preparing the body for *I'll be more prepared next time*, as a lowered sense of self-worth is the result of defeat in the CA phase of the shock. A victory would result in the opposite of a lowering of self-worth, nor would it likely produce shock, but rather exuberance.

Osteoporosis then is the result of a prolonged unresolved self-devaluation conflict. The bone is preparing to become stronger, but the resolution, that would create a stronger bone does one of two things. Either it doesn't occur, and the bone continues to decalcify, which doctors would then notice in routine physical examinations or is delayed long enough so that when healing does occur, the bone is more vulnerable to breaking. During healing, the periosteum, a membrane that covers the bone and provides, among other things, stabilization, stretches due to the increased fluids at the repair site (all healing occurs in a fluid medium), reducing its support effectiveness. If this happens after a prolonged CA period of a self-worth DHS, the bone will break more readily, and the resulting visit to the emergency room will likely include a diagnosis of osteoporosis, and a bleak prognosis.

To answer the location questions posed in the *Mainstream* section of this chapter, GNM relates hips to a DHS associated with heavy continuous demands, mid to lower spine with a devaluation conflict that strikes at the core of one's self, and shoulders with having a devaluation conflict that stems from a failed relationship. GNM has mapped most every part of our structure to a specific conflict.

Menopause is a milestone event in a woman's life, especially in mothers. It signals the end of the capacity to bring new life into the world, and for many, children are leaving the nest. A myriad of symptoms often accompanies this passage, many of which are stark reminders of aging: thinning of the hair, weight gain, dry skin, and loss of breast mass. It is easy to see how these symptoms could result in a loss of self-worth. If the reality of menopause is enough to trigger a DHS, there will be no resolution to the conflict other than acceptance, as age is not reversible, and the reminders of that fact will only increase with time. Recall that earlier in this chapter, I pointed out that roughly 50% of women suffer osteoporosis. Now I'd like to introduce you to another tidbit: nearly half of all women in the USA never have children.[88] Pure coincidence? No overlap? You decide.

Arthritis involves this same self-devaluation conflict manifesting itself in joints, so not as *deep*, not as strong as with bone. In cases of hanging-healing (see *Allergies:Maverick* chapter), the joint will alternate between decalcification and calcification, eventually deforming the joint due to repeated incomplete buildup of callus. Mainstream medicine has labeled this condition as chronic arthritis.

Teeth are specialized bones. They enable biting and chewing. Literal or figurative conflicts involving not being able to bite (dentin), or not being allowed to bite (enamel) result in the standard bone pattern of decalcification, followed by calcification upon conflict resolution. Both of these conflicts involve reigning in the desire to bite (in humans this mostly occurs in the abstract sense), with pain serving as a compelling reminder. Once the conflict is resolved, slow re-calcification is painless. GNM maintains that tooth decay is unrelated to sugary foods, or bacterial acids. Note that the normal pH of children's saliva is slightly alkaline (7.5)[89]. Should not this decidedly non-acidic environment, which is necessary for the activation of the starch-digesting enzyme amylase, neutralize much, if not all the acid formed by bacteria present in the mouth? How does this data align with the fact that globally, 60-90 percent of all school children have dental cavities?[90]

Audit

Hundreds of millions of dollars are spent in the USA alone every year to *combat* diseases of this nature. This has been happening for many decades, yet brittle bones still plague the elderly, arthritis robs millions of their dexterity, and billions of teeth are filled or pulled annually. These particular health problems are either fiendishly complicated to correct or prevent by their nature, or the conventional methods of doing so are ineffective.

Dr. Hamer's research into this area has yielded a remarkably cohesive understanding of structural health problems. To summarize his conclusions, the hard tissue of our bodies provides structure. Shocks

Healthcare

that affect this structure are dealt with by attempting to make the structure stronger at the expense of weight, and thus agility (a stronger, denser structure is heavier). Unlike most SBSs, the biological advantage here is realized at the end of PCL-B (last part of the healing phase), as creating a denser bone, requires Nature to first ulcerate, or deconstruct the existing bone mass, rebuilding with a *tighter weave*, so to speak, after this preparation is finished (CL). This category of disease primarily affects those on the ends of either side of the physical prime of life, where perceived structural weakness is more keenly felt. Ignorance of cause and societal circumstances play significant roles in the chronic reality of these problems. Knowledge is the antidote for this first reason, and is useful in overcoming some of the negative health affects of the second.

The good news here is that adding knowledge does not cost very much. The alternative, currently the status quo, is more of the same, measured in enormous cost, futility, and pain.

Brain

This chapter deals with disorders of the brain other than cancer (see *Cancer* chapter).

Dementia has been described as a decline in mental abilities or cognitive functions. It usually occurs in the elderly, but is not unknown in people as young as 30.

Stroke is either a blocked or ruptured blood vessel that feeds the brain.

Huntington's disease (HD) is a fatal genetic disorder of the brain. It is marked by a breakdown of nerve cells.

Migraines present as incapacitating headaches and other neurological symptoms. They are often accompanied by extreme sensitivity to light and sound and may lead to nausea and vomiting.

Organizations

Stroke is the second leading cause of death worldwide[91], and fifth leading cause of death in the United States. The leading private medical organization dedicated to preventing stroke is part of a larger organization dedicated to solving the problem of heart disease.

The leading medical charitable organization dedicated to eradicating Huntington's disease (HD) was founded in 1967.[92] In 50 years, they have grown to 54 volunteer-led chapters and affiliates across the United States with a headquarters in New York City. Their revenue for 2016 was reported as $8,578,920.[93]

Another such organization reportedly donates $100 million[94] per year for HD research, largely to develop drugs to slow the progress and improve the lives of the victims of HD.

The leading charity seeking a solution to Alzheimer's disease[95] shares a similar goal for their target illness, promotes overall brain health to reduce the threat of dementia, and provides a support and care network for all those affected by this dreaded disease. They have been doing so for 37 years, having been founded in 1980. They currently have 271 local chapters throughout the United States, and a yearly revenue (for 2016) of just under $178 million.[96]

The US federal government also funds research into brain disorders. Their funding, as usual, dwarfs private contributions (see *Appendix*). Not surprisingly, these efforts focus mainly on allopathic protocols.

Mainstream Theory

Mainstream medicine acknowledges two types of stroke. Ischemic strokes are the result of an obstructed blood vessel supplying the brain. Hemorrhagic strokes result from ruptured blood vessels in the brain. Both result in the death of brain cells, which depending on the amount of damage and location, can prove fatal.

Surgeons have long known that it is not uncommon to find arterial walls coated with fatty deposits, a condition known within allopathy as atherosclerosis. They observe that sometimes, these deposits break loose, travel in the blood vessels until they lodge in a smaller section, creating a blockage. Blockages can also occur from mobile blood clots. This obstruction deprives the cells that are served by this blood vessel of the oxygen and nutrients present in the blood, resulting in the death of those cells. When it happens in the brain, symptoms can occur in the bodily functions controlled by the stricken portion of the brain.

There are 10,000 miles[97] (6.3 billion inches) of blood vessels (mostly capillaries) in an average adult human body, and roughly 400 miles[98] (just over 25.3 million inches) in the brain alone, which averages about 80 cubic inches in volume. Simple division yields a figure of 312,500 inches (5 miles) of blood vessels per cubic inch of brain matter. In order for any blockage to act in the manner described above, it must obstruct a major artery, one that is not part of a redundancy network, so-called collateral circulation, such as the Circle of Willis[99] in the brain.

It really should come as no surprise that Nature has built redundancy into such an important responsibility as feeding brain cells. Think of it kind of like a (one way) road system. Roads are seldom dangling branches, especially in crowded areas (your brain) like cities. They are usually joined, so that there is more than one way of getting to your destination. If one road is blocked, for whatever reason, you can typically still get where you are going, by taking an alternate route.

Hemorrhagic strokes,[100] which account for 13% of all strokes are responsible for 40% of stroke deaths. A hemorrhagic stroke is one where a blood vessel ruptures. Since the skull, being bone, doesn't expand, the continuous pressure from the heart is now transferred to the wound. This pressure, now pressing on brain tissue, can cut off blood flow in nearby vessels, starving, and eventually killing, brain cells. If the affected area controls vital functions, it is easy to see how this can be catastrophic. The standard answer to why these ruptures occur is high blood pressure and atherosclerosis.

The consensus mainstream medical opinion is that Huntington's disease is a fatal genetic disease that has no cure.[101] There is also no effective treatment to stall the progression of the disease. In 1993, it was reported that a gene complicit in HD was discovered. Since then, all effort has been made leveraging that discovery in developing treatments, and hopefully a cure. That was 24 years ago. There is apparently still no effective treatment, and still no cure. Nor could I find any hint of either. There is also no mention how the gene was changed to cause HD. An entire science, epigenetics, is showing that genes are not static, that they change, or are changed (by the brain?), in response to outside stimulus. If this science is correct, and the evidence is compelling,[102] the pursuit of a cure using gene modification faces a steep uphill struggle, as the target can apparently move. Identifying the stimulus that causes the change, thereby illuminating a reverse path, will perhaps yield better results. A private HD research foundation has made it their mission[103] to slow the progression of HD through the development of therapeutics. Such is the devastation of this disease that even to only slow its march is considered success. It appears that the current allopathic state of the art does not include anything more ambitious at this time.

Dementia is a broad category[104] of mental diminishment, most often caused by Alzheimer's disease (50-70%), and vascular issues, such as mini-strokes (15-20%). Allopaths have identified an accumulation of a protein called beta amyloid in the areas of the brain controlling memory and cognition in patients suffering from Alzheimer's disease, and have concluded that this buildup is the cause of the disease. What causes the buildup is not well understood. There is no effective treatment for either Alzheimer's disease or mini-strokes in allopathy[105] and therefore, no effective treatment for dementia. Statements such as *irreversible*, and, *cannot be cured* typify the attitude of mainstream medicine toward this condition. Perhaps these indications of a dead-end road ought to warrant a sea change in the direction of medical research in this field, as Alzheimer's disease is currently the 6th leading cause of death in the USA, but is predicted to surge as the baby boom generation ages.[106]

Recalling a highly practical, essentially no-cost, protocol from the chapter *The Alternative Solutions*, water, or more specifically, dehydration, is linked quite strongly to dementia. Care-home doctors and nurses have noticed that dehydration can share symptoms with dementia or aggravate a dementious state. Rehydrating a patient can often abate the symptoms thereby resulting in a better quality of life.[107] I don't presume that dementia = dehydration, only that it might help for all of us, and especially the elderly, to drink enough water. Dr. Batmanghelidj would no doubt concur.

Migraine headaches are the third most prevalent (affecting an estimated 1 billion people worldwide) and sixth most disabling disease in the world.[108] This results in a staggering estimate of $36 billion in healthcare costs and lost productivity each year in the US alone. The Migraine Research Foundation takes a refreshing position on their target, but as yet, offers no cure. They admit that they don't understand what causes migraines, but recognize that therein lies the key to developing effective treatments. This rare acknowledgment is hopefully directing research in that direction. Whatever lack of success in overcoming migraines is not from a lack of trying. The earliest recorded migraines were in ancient Egypt, circa 1200 BC. True to form, the earliest allopathic success came in the late 1930s, with the discovery of a vasoconstriction drug to relieve symptoms.

Maverick Theory

The brain is a central organ in the GNM view of disease. It, like the psyche, is involved in every DHS, as a conflict shock will manifest simultaneously on the psyche, the brain, and the affected organ. We cannot directly measure the psyche, but thanks to technology, science has no such trouble with the brain. Per GNM theory and observation, an SBS is triggered in the brain at the time of the shock, which manifests as a target ring configuration, or lesion (HH). The HH will remain in this form throughout the conflict-active (CA) phase, only undergoing changes upon conflict resolution (CL), which are visible on a CT scan, as the healing phase progresses (evidence of the brain repairing itself). During the first part of the healing phase (PCL-A), edema (fluid) accumulates to protect the repair (in both brain and organ). This fluid is expelled during the relatively brief epileptoid crisis (EC) phase. In the brain, this expulsion can press against critical nerve pathways, resulting in heart attack (as pressure interrupts the heart rhythm centers [left for arterial fibrillation], and [right for arrhythmia or cardiac arrest]), strokes, asthma attacks, and epileptic seizures depending on HH location. During the last part of the healing phase (PCL-B), glial tissue fills the brain HH area, enabling the reconnection of damaged neurons. Allopathic oncology identifies this phenomenon as a brain tumor.

GNM gives a different reason for cerebral aneurysms (hemorrhagic stroke). Instead of atherosclerosis, GNM proposes that repeated scarring in the healing process described above due to relapses (new DHS or tracks), results in the tissue becoming more rigid, and therefore more prone to rupture in the physical stress of the EC. Since many of the symptoms of stroke[109] involve movement, GNM associates them with motor conflicts (see *Central Nervous System* chapter for further discussion of motor [self-devaluation] conflicts), and EC complications when pressure disrupts motor centers in the brain.

Huntington's Disease (HD) primarily affects motor faculties, as do multiple sclerosis, ALS, and other similar maladies (see more in *Central Nervous System* chapter). Allopathy sees them as distinct diseases or infections, as the altered cells are in different areas of the body (in the case of HD, the brain). GNM classifies all of these as part of the play-dead survival reflex commonly observed in prey animals. All of these *diseases* in humans are usually degenerative, that is, they most often get worse with time. Some are fatal. GNM explains this as hanging-active or hanging-healing, where the sight of a malfunctioning body part and the accompanying dismal medical prognosis, lead the patient into an endless loop of conflicts, which never have a chance to either fully resolve or heal. The SBSs are never allowed to exit. According to GNM, all these diseases share a similar conflict, one of being stuck, of being physically or figuratively unable to escape, to move. The conflict is one of self-devaluation, but not as intense as one that would affect the bones. As such, the CA phase is marked by ulceration, followed, unless hanging-active, by cell restoration and repair. A hanging-healing of this conflict often occurs in the EC phase, which is aptly named crisis.

GNM has observed that memory loss always accompanies separation conflicts. This occurs in the CA phase, as Nature tries to lessen the shock by blocking the painful memory of separation. Typically, the conflict, and thus the memory loss, are short term. Long-term separation, however, can lead to dementia. Mainstream medicine corroborates this by recognizing that short-term memories are the ones affected in early dementia; as dementia progresses (DHS doesn't resolve, or tracks interrupt the healing), longer-term memories are altered as well.

Migraine headaches result from DHSs that involve danger and powerlessness. They begin in the PCL phase and affect the thyroid duct relay and the branchial arch relay in the frontal area of the brain.

Healthcare

Migraines become most intense during the EC phase, as the edema surrounding the affected brain relay is expelled. A KCTS (see *Kidneys and Bladder* chapter) can multiply the edema, amplifying the migraine symptoms. Chronic migraines are the result of tracks, which can take the form of sensory stimuli, stress, and other migraine triggers.

Audit

A leading medical organization[110] estimates that roughly 80,000 new cases of primary brain tumor will be diagnosed in 2017, adding to the current US total of 700,000 patients. The cost of brain surgery[111] ranges from $50,000 to roughly $700,000. Do the math: worst case $500 billion, best case $35 billion, if everyone underwent surgery. Even then, there would be no guarantee that they would only need one. Add $4 billion to $56 billion yearly to that total to cover new cases.

Migraines add upwards of $17 billion[112] annually to the total. Dementia adds $157 billion[113] annually and strokes another $34 billion[114] per year.

The US federal government spends billions of tax dollars every year on brain issues. Private organizations spend hundreds of millions more researching cures.

Conventional treatment of brain diseases is unsurprisingly expensive, as the brain is extraordinarily complex. A large piece of the pie is spent on rehabilitation costs or aftercare. All of this seemingly proceeds from an uncertain comprehension of clear cause. Couple this with similar stories for other diseases to produce a textbook definition of unsustainability. Throughout this book, I argue for understanding cause; numbers like this demand it.

Cancer

Cancer as an umbrella term for diseases in which rogue cells multiply out of control, sometimes invading other tissues in the body where they continue to proliferate. The professional study of cancer is called oncology.

Organization

The preeminent cancer charity organization[115] was founded in 1913. They have focused on cancer research for more than a century now, and are indeed, one of the largest such medical organizations in the US. They combine research, education, advocacy, and service to improve the lives of cancer victims and their loved ones. Their goal is the elimination of cancer.[116] They are highly organized into 11 geographical divisions with 900+ offices throughout the United States. Their expenses for 2015 were $940,543,000,[117] the bulk of which is funded by private donations.

Funding for cancer research at the US federal government level is even higher (see *Appendix*), having exploded upward in 1971 when President Nixon declared war on cancer. Roughly 600,000 people in the USA die from the disease yearly, placing it second on the leading cause of death list.

Both of these organizations focus on the allopathic medical paradigm in their research. Since allopathy is the dominant therapeutic approach used in hospitals today to treat cancer, I feel secure judging the efficacy of allopathy in treating cancer using government provided statistics.[118]

The good news is that survival rates are increasing; the bad news is that statistics on being cancer free are not to be had. It is therefore impossible for me to tell how much of this increase is due solely to advances in early detection (a strength of allopathy), raising the question of whether a 6 or even 7-year survival rate chart should replace the current 5-year survival standard.

Mainstream Theory

In their search for a solution to cancer, what approach has been the primary focus of allopathic oncology? Chemotherapy, radiation, and surgery. How has that panned out? How do allopaths, or more specifically, in this case, allopathic oncologists, measure success?

The go-to allopathic measure of success for cancer treatment is the five-year survival rate statistic. That is, from the time you are diagnosed, the question is asked: what is your chance of survival five years down the road? Notice the glaring hole in this measure; it says nothing of whether you still have cancer.

In any other measure in this life, if you identify something unwanted and target it for removal, success is measured by the absence of that target. If you have a termite infestation in your house, your solution is considered a success when all of the termites are gone, not whether your house is still standing five years on. If you are trying to launch a communication satellite, and your rockets keep failing, success is achieved by actually placing a satellite in orbit, not by merely managing to avoid bankruptcy for five years. Why is cancer treatment different?

Cancer

Is it because cause is uncertain? That should cast serious doubt on the primacy of the target. Is it because cancer sometimes returns after so-called successful treatment?[119] Putting aside cases of poisoning (not category F), one possible explanation for this return is that Nature has a reason for producing those cells. Since her primary function is survival, are the two somehow related? And since this treatment is toxic to all cells, healthy or not,[120] I have to wonder how responsible this protocol is for cancer mortality.

One of the goals of this approach to cancer treatment is early detection. Since technology is a strength of Western medicine, better imaging should help doctors push the survival rate envelope in a positive direction. It is assumed that if a tumor is detected while still small, it can more easily be defeated, but since success is not measured in this paradigm by the defeat of cancer, but by a 5-year survival rate, the main result of early detection is pushing the curve left. What I mean by that is a typical survival rate curve looks something like this, where the chance of survival drops as time advances from the initial cancer diagnosis. I am extrapolating this generic survival curve (they all resemble an exponential decay curve) for years 6 and 7, since standard research shows 5-year data only.

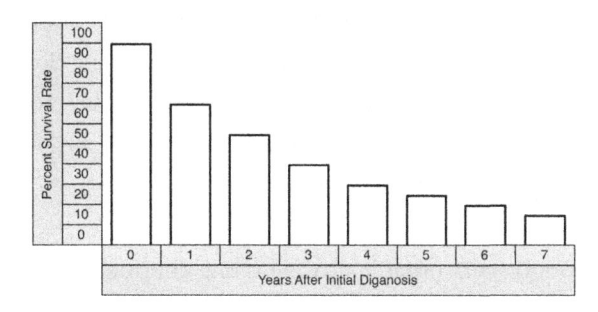

If I paint a 5-year window onto this chart (heavy border below), and then shift initial detections 2 years earlier (light border), you get a clearer picture. Year-0 (highest survival rate) in the heavy chart is year-2

Healthcare

for the light chart. Success rates for years zero and one are only available if the cancer is detected earlier. Put another way, if you wait two years after the earliest possible detection, your yearly survival rates are lower than what they would have been.

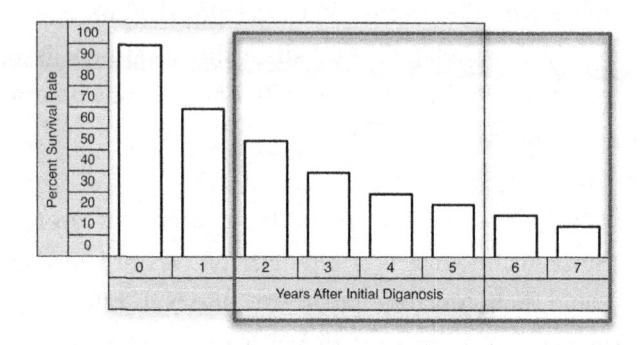

This does not take into account that people die as they age in general, nor does it distinguish between different types of cancers, but the trend is less than optimistic.

I fashioned my hypothetical graphs above based on a study of actual 5-year cancer survival rate graphs from an extensive network of hospitals dedicated to the treatment of cancer.[121] A grim story unfolded as I viewed their published 5-year survival rate graphs of many cancers (albeit with metastases, or cancers in multiple locations).[122] These charts help explain the annual number of cancer deaths. Some are more optimistic than others. All trend seemingly inexorably toward death, differing only in the steepness of their slope. Metastatic cancer, also known as stage IV, offers the least hope of survival.

I have no doubt this organization is using the methods they employ to their fullest potential. It is clear to me they are passionate about helping people regain their health. In addition to treatment, they offer a wide range of support for cancer patients and their loved ones, but searching their site for the cause of cancer left me with no answers other than the standard ones where statistical risk factors are cited. As I have stated before, I am of the opinion that if you don't understand the cause of a particular disease, then you are trusting your recovery from that disease to dumb luck. I hope I can do better, and I'm guessing so do you.

Since cancer charities fund much of the research into the treatments mainstream oncologists implement, I thought perhaps they could provide answers as to cause. What I found surprised me, though in hindsight, given cancer statistics, I really could have guessed. Searching for *what causes xyz cancer* on one such site, I found no definitive answers. There were many sections dedicated to this question, but no clear answers that I could see. Their explanations of the root(s) of this disease seemed to me depressingly repetitive. Below are a series of links from their site to specific cancers (not xyz) so that you can draw your own conclusions. I have no interest in pasting their words into this book, as one can always hope they may change for the better (which this book, once printed, cannot).

- Ovarian cancer.[123]
- Lung cancer.[124]
- Liver cancer.[125]
- Bone cancer.[126]
- Cancers of the brain and spinal cord.[127]
- Colorectal cancer.[128]
- Stomach cancer.[129]
- Pancreatic cancer.[130]
- Breast cancer.[131]
- Melanoma (skin cancer).[132]
- Testicular cancer.[133]
- Childhood leukemia (cancer of the blood).[134]
- Acute lymphocytic leukemia.[135]
- Oral cavity or oropharyngeal cancer.[136]

Healthcare

To summarize, in every case on this list as of 2017, this organization is uncertain of cause. I found no instance of *we estimate we are X% to our goal of understanding what causes this cancer*, and certainly no instances of *we've got this one figured out* – not one. Phrases such as *the exact cause*, or *don't know*, or *can't say*, or *partially understood*, are in my opinion, just other ways of expressing frustration at what appears to me to be fundamental causal ignorance.

Perhaps you feel I'm being harsh, so let me dissect one of these answers as to cause. To me, they are unfortunately all variations of the same theme, so I'll randomly pick one: bone cancer. Reviewing their conclusion, do they mean that the exact cause of some bone cancers is known? If that were so, I would expect to see words to the effect of *If you have xyz bone cancer, we have got that completely figured out. Not to worry, just visit your oncologist, and he'll fix you right up.* There is no statement remotely resembling that on their bone cancer web pages, so I'll conclude that they don't mean that. From my perspective, *most* is a distraction. It makes for a softer, but less accurate version of the slightly shorter sentence, *The exact cause of bone cancer is unknown.* The other curious word in that statement is *exact*. Do they mean that *The partial cause of most bone cancers is known*? I believe that is what they mean. This organization has much to say about risk factors associated with cancer. Genetics, environment, associated health problems are all implicated in some patients with cancer, but rarely in those with bone cancer. So here is again, for the most part, another soft sell. Why not just tell it plain? Is it because then, the sentence would read *The cause of bone cancer is unknown*? By applying this Socratic type of method to any answer as to cause from the above list of links, I arrive at a similar basic statement; you may not. Taken together, these statements distill for me to: *the cause of cancer is unknown,* a decidedly pessimistic conclusion if you maintain (as I do) that an understanding of cause is a critical component in your return to health.

While I'm on bone cancer, bones contain marrow at their core, which is responsible for the creation of blood cells, platelets, bone, cartilage, and fat. A major disease originating in bone marrow is leukemia, which in acute cases is characterized by an abundance of immature white blood cells (leukoblasts). Acute leukemias apparently respond positively to chemotherapy. Popular chemotherapy drugs for these types of cancer are powerful bone marrow suppressors,[137] so it's not surprising that leukoblast production (as well as every other cell marrow produces) is drastically curtailed in this assault. Well, that can't be a long-term solution, as bone marrow is essential for life. So what happens after the drug is stopped? It is hoped that the bone marrow recovers, sans cancer.[138] This strategy, though far more serious, reminds me a little of a computer reboot: if your laptop is freaking out, and you don't know why, cycle power – that will give you a clean slate, and hopefully the glitches will be gone when it starts up again. Maybe, but you really don't know what happened to cause the problem, so if rebooting doesn't do the trick, it's time for another strategy – off to the computer repair ace, who will pinpoint the cause of the problem and eliminate or replace it, and voilà, you're back in business. For leukemia, so called second-line strategies are more drugs, which again target symptoms, for as you just saw, cause is unclear. This is just another example of why understanding cause is really not optional. Here's food for thought: since both of these cancers seem to originate in bone, are they somehow related? Mainstream oncology views leukemia as a blood cancer and says no.[139]

There are many other cancers, but I think the point is made. If the cancer you are interested in is not on this list, you should be able to find it from one of the previous links. Allopaths have studied the heck out of cancer for 100 years, directing unimaginable effort, time, and money at this problem, but are still uncertain as to cause. Their dedication to eradicating this disease from the human experience is not in question. Their progress in all other aspects of cancer care is impressive. My question though, to me the root of this issue, is, what causes cancer? For that question mainstream medicine does not offer clear, unambiguous guidance. Maybe no such answers are to be had, or maybe some base assumptions of mainstream oncology are just plain wrong.

The 5-year survival charts with the worst prognoses, the steepest slopes, are for patients diagnosed with distant, or metastatic cancers. This cancer phenomenon is explained by allopathy as cells having somehow broken loose from an original cancer site and traveling to other parts of the body via either the bloodstream, or the lymph system. These traveling cells then inexplicably stop, against the never ceasing flow of blood or lymph, attach themselves somehow to the vessel in which they are traveling, pass through this vessel, again somehow, without springing multiple leaks and finally establish themselves at this new body site to continue their unchecked growth, albeit transformed now, somehow, into the cells of their new site. It appears that this explanation requires cancer cells to possess intelligence, extra-functional capabilities and bi-directional transformative powers.

Well, that is one explanation. That there are cancerous cells in more than one location in these patients is a fact. That this occurred via the mechanism proposed by allopathic oncology is a theory. If true, there should be rational explanations for the following questions:

- Why is donated blood not screened for cancer cells?[140]
- Why does the blood/brain barrier not stop cancer cells from crossing into the brain?
- Why do so-called brain tumors rarely[141] metastasize?
- Why is angiosarcoma (cancer of the cells that line blood and lymph vessels) exceedingly rare[142] (2% of 0.7% < 0.02%) when presumably, they are in near constant contact with cancer cells in a patient with metastasis?

- What is the mechanism that causes differentiated cells that happen to turn cancerous into undifferentiated cells (similar to stem cells) so that they may take hold in a different part of the body and re-differentiate?
  - If this is not the case, how do liver cells, for example, take root in the lung to form a lung tumor? Presumably, lung tumors consist of lung cells.

It has been estimated[143] that 90% of all cancer deaths occur in patients with metastatic cancers, and yet, only 5% of cancer research funds are spent on this phenomenon. Why?

Alternative Theory

TCM treats cancer according to symptoms.[144] It is generally a twofold approach, with one hand attempting to indirectly address the disease by fortifying a patient's general health, while the other targets the cancer directly. Herbs, acupuncture, and acupressure attempt to restore balance to the body. Thousands of years of trial and error have yielded a remarkably diverse and effective natural pharmacopeia of ways to balance yin and yang. TCM identifies the primary culprit in cancer progression as toxic heat. Herbs are the main tool used in its removal from the body.

Ayurveda[145] sees cancer as an opportunistic growth caused by low enzyme reserves and primarily seeks to implement a preventive strategy.

Homeopathy is not considered a primary therapy for cancer. It is often used in conjunction with other natural therapies to great success. There are three basic approaches to homeopathic cancer treatment. One strategy is to target tumors directly. Here, homeopaths select remedies based on the image of the tumor, either administering them orally as is standard practice, or sometimes injecting them directly in or near the tumor site. In addition, homeopathics are used to assist the body to eliminate the toxins present in cancers. The kidneys, the lymph and the liver are prime targets for strengthening. Still another approach is constitutional homeopathy. This strategy attempts to right the body at a holistic level, enabling it to remove the cancer more effectively.

Naturopathy[146] represents a vast array of potential medical modalities. As such, it is difficult to generalize about a naturopathic approach to cancer. However, it is safe to say that a large part of the strategy is as a co-treatment to allopathic methods, seeking to lessen the effects of that treatment through natural means.

An experienced physician in any of these modalities will seek to lessen the fear and anxiety all too present in recently diagnosed cancer patients, proceeding from the assumption that these emotions can overwhelm, and as such are hardly beneficial on the patient's road to recovery. Such emotions typically trigger a fight or flight response, neither of which is practical in the face of the threat of cancer. You can't run away from your cancer, and fighting your own cells is nonsensical. I realize that a standard response to most health threats is *to fight*, which meshes well with the mainstream jargon of waging war on disease, but in this context, *don't give up or hang in there* are more accurate descriptions of the instinct.

A comprehensive collection of alternative cancer protocols can be found at www.cancertutor.com, where scores of alternative cancer treatments are discussed and dissected.

Cancer

Maverick Theory

The revelation that is German New Medicine (GNM) was the result of an investigation by Dr. Ryke Geerd Hamer into his testicular cancer, which was diagnosed shortly after the death of his son Dirk to a bullet wound. These two seemingly disparate events are actually integrally linked; shock can lead to cancer, which incidentally is the First Biological Law of GNM, (The Iron Rule of Cancer). What Dr. Hamer discovered caused him to lose his medical license (by not complying with mainstream oncological methods), be thrown into prison (accused of practicing medicine without a license), and have to retreat into exile (to continue his discovery of GNM without harassment). Cancer was at the core of this discovery, so as you might expect, GNM has much to say about cancer.

Allopathic oncology defines cancer as out of control cell growth.[147] GNM proposes a reason for why cells proliferate, and strongly disagrees that there is no control. They propose, via the Second Biological Law (Law of 2 Phases), that the body rids itself of these extra cells when they are no longer needed, or rebuilds cells that were initially ulcerated, which is when one typically becomes aware of them. This is a coherent explanation as to why oncologists mostly see rotting, not healthy, extra cells, or cells regenerating at a truly rapid pace, seemingly out of control. According to GNM, this is all part of an evolutionary plan to ensure the survival of the individual, a position that to a cancer patient or survivor ignorant of GNM must seem absurd. Please bear with me.

Five biological laws define GNM. Refer to the previous chapter entitled *The Maverick Solution* for an explanation of each and to several key acronyms. GNM proposes that cancer is a class of reactions to perceived shock. In a nutshell, according to GNM, cancer is a response to a subconscious perceived need for a (mostly temporary) change in body functionality. In the 2 phases of the SBS, either an organ cell loss or cell gain (based on HH location in the brain), creates the desired change in the first phase, followed upon conflict resolution with its reverse, cell gain or loss, in the second phase. Large tumors are often the result of prolonged conflicts, conflict relapses, or tracks, leading to either a hanging-active or hanging-healing situation. I will use a few hypothetical examples to illustrate.

Breast Cancer (Adenoid Mammary Carcinoma). GNM recognizes, and has explanations for three types of breast cancer. This particular one (milk-producing glands) occurs in response to a nest-worry conflict, which is a form of attack conflict. The HH (CT scan ring pattern) can be seen in the cerebellum, indicating initial cell gain, which can often be seen as one or more lumps in the breast. These will remain, producing more milk until the conflict has been resolved, whereupon the extra cells are decomposed by tuberculosis bacteria. If no TB is present (due to antibiotics), the tumor encapsulates and stays. Sharp stabbing pains while healing are due to the scarring process, which ends with a depression (hole) where the tumor once was.

Examples of this type of DHS (conflict shock) could involve a child (a biological extension of the mother) running into oncoming traffic, or falling and cracking their head on the pavement. The resulting increase in milk-producing cells provides more nourishment for a stricken child, speeding their recovery. This SBS (2-phase reaction to DHS) is present in all maternal mammals, not just humans, and presumably hails from a time before emergency rooms.

Cancer of the Small Intestine occurs in response to an indigestible-morsel conflict (actual morsel or figurative, as in not being able to digest a morsel; anger with family, friends, colleagues). The HH is centered in the brainstem indicating initial cell gain, which if prolonged, will grow enough to be classified as a tumor. This evolutionary response results in more intestinal cells for better absorption of food and is generally not noticeable in the first phase of the SBS (conflict-active [CA]) unless the conflict is so intense (or prolonged) that the cell growth obstructs the passage of food, in which case emergency surgery may be required. Once the conflict is resolved (CL), fungi and bacteria will decompose the tumor(s), and the patient can expect pain (a common symptom accompanying swelling), bloody stool and the passing of tumor remains.

Pulmonary Lung Cancer (Adenocarcinoma) is always the result of a death-fright conflict shock (example: cancer diagnosis shock perceived as a death sentence, which is why lung cancer is a common metastatic[148]). As always, this shock (DHS) is subjective; for a death-fright conflict, a person only needs to perceive that the event is potentially fatal. The HH is centered in the cerebellum indicating initial cell gain. In biological terms the death panic is equated with an inability to breathe, causing the alveoli to multiply, possibly forming a tumor (a function of conflict intensity/duration). This growth is not painful and will continue until conflict resolution (CL). Any extra cells (tumors) will then be decomposed by mycobacteria such as tubercular bacteria (provided they are present). These tumors become caseated and are coughed out, and all that will remain are caverns (holes in the lung). If no TB is available (due to antibiotics), the tumor encapsulates and stays.

These examples are short peeks into three common forms of cancer that have often proved fatal when treated with standard oncological methods.[149] When cause is not even acknowledged in the treatment, due to ignorance, all that is left for the doctor, is to attack symptoms. If GNM is correct, this is a battle against Nature, which is employing all means to keep you alive. Ideally, a doctor should aid Nature.

GNM has investigated most forms of cancer, as recorded by allopathic oncology. From the affected organ functionality, it has noted the control

Healthcare

center(s) for that organ in the brain as determined by embryology. This location determines whether initial cell gain or loss is indicated. Once that is ascertained, logical scenarios of how such loss/gain would benefit the organ are assessed. From there, it is often a small step to identify typical real-world conflicts that could trigger such behavior. Another hypothetical example will hopefully clarify:

A. Cancerous tumors are known to grow in the liver.[150]
B. The brainstem controls the liver (the cerebral cortex controls the liver's bile ducts), which indicates initial liver cell gain by an SBS, to be followed by cell loss once the conflict has been resolved.
C. How might more liver cells (initial body response to conflict shock [DHS]) temporarily biologically benefit an individual to aid them in overcoming this shock?
D. The responsibility of the cells of the liver includes the metabolism of proteins, fats, and carbohydrates. In other words, the liver plays a crucial role in converting the food you eat into energy and building blocks that your body needs to survive.
E. If you have more such liver cells, your liver would conceivably be more efficient in metabolizing what food you do manage to eat. Such increased functionality would be very handy in times of famine to squeeze more nutrition out of every meal, but be unnecessary given adequate access to food.
F. Let us call a *fear of starvation event* a *starvation conflict*. How might a starvation conflict occur? Remember, a DHS is subjective; different people will react uniquely to the same event. Here are a few potential conflict examples:
- Any prolonged economic hardship, introducing uncertainty as to how you will pay for your next meal.

Cancer

- Any period of prolonged nausea, which would hamper your ability to keep down food, such as is common with certain kinds of chemotherapy.[151]
- Damage to stomach or intestines (cancer surgery, combat damage, accidental poisoning, etc.), causing doubt as to whether you will be able to digest enough food to live.

G. If a starvation conflict occurs, hopefully, it is temporary. Its resolution will reverse the cell gain. The loss will be accompanied by pain and swelling, as all cell growth occurs in a fluid medium, which will cause pressure, often against nerves. This discomfort will be proportional to the length and intensity of the conflict. It may very well command attention.

H. If it does, that will most probably elicit a visit to a doctor, who may notice (from a biopsy) cells in the process of destruction. As GNM is largely unknown in the medical community, the doctor will most probably express concern, and suspect cancer. The initial presence of a healthy cluster of cells is water under the bridge and simply not imagined.

I. Nor will a connection be made to a starvation conflict and the subsequent resolution thereof.

J. Any CT scan made of the brain in search of metastasis will likely show a healing HH (ring pattern) in the liver parenchyma relay in the brainstem. If noticed at all, it will likely be dismissed as an artifact or possibly raise concern as a potential brain tumor. A liver scan may also show an HH.

K. If the patient interprets this diagnosis as a terrifying potential death sentence, another SBS could be triggered by this new shock (DHS). This time it could very likely occur in the lungs (alveoli), the organ location of all death-fright conflicts, and culminate in a subsequent diagnosis of lung

cancer through metastasis. This second diagnosis could lead to further DHSs. Knowledge of what is happening is required to abort this deadly downward spiral.
L. Ignorance of how cancer occurs, that it is not, as Dr. Hamer noted "senseless disturbances to be repaired by aspiring sorcerers," even that your body is reacting to your ignorance and fear, are all things that depress the slopes of the grim 5-year survival graphs published by allopathic oncological institutions.

Common cancer inducing conflicts and their target organs are listed[152] below. See *The Maverick Solution* chapter for more information on these conflict categories. This list is incomplete and only intended to show that GNM has offered an explanation for the cause of many cancers identified by mainstream oncology. I have dedicated this short chapter to cancer; the topic requires several full-length books to do it justice, not to mention an expertise which I lack. The reference section of this book contains sources where you can explore in deeper detail.

Morsel conflicts
- *Colon* Unable to absorb or digest (evolutionary holdover)
- *Esophagus (upper 2/3)* Unwilling to swallow
- *Esophagus (lower 1/3)* Unable to swallow
- *Intestines* Unable to absorb or digest
- *Liver* Starvation
- *Lung* Death-fright
- *Pancreas* Unable to absorb or digest
- *Rectum* Unable to eliminate
- *Stomach (large curvature)* Unable to stomach, unable to digest
- *Thyroid* Unable to grab or release

Conflict of insufficient peristalsis

- The smooth musculature of intestine, uterus, heart and blood vessels do experience cell growth, but as far as I can tell, allopathy does not recognize this as cancer.

Attack Conflicts
- *Breast glands* Nest worry. Nonsexual argument with partner
- *Corium skin (dermis)* Literal or perceived attack

Self-devaluation Conflicts
- *Adrenal cortex* Wrong direction, gone astray; AKA Addison's disease
- *Bone* Severe loss of self-worth; Leukemia in SBS healing phase
- *Kidneys* Too much water or fluid
- *Lymph glands* Moderate loss of self-worth
- *Prostate and Uterus* Procreation or mating
- *Testes and Ovaries* Loss of child

Territorial Conflicts
- *Bladder mucosa and Urethra* Marking
- *Bronchials* Fear of territorial intrusion.
- *Cervix* Sexual
- *Gall bladder* Anger (male) or identity (female) conflict
- *Larynx* Fear (male) or scare-fright (female) conflict
- *Pancreatic ducts* Anger
- *Stomach (small curvature)* Anger (male) or identity (female) conflict

Separation Conflicts
- *Breast milk duct* Child or partner separation (torn from my breast)
- *Skin (epidermis)* Longing for touch or revulsion at touch

Audit

Cancer is a dreaded word. It invokes that dread largely because mainstream medical science's effort to stop it is all too often ineffective in preventing a terrible, lingering death for the patient. Cancer is the second leading cause of death in the USA. That reality culminates in panic, justifying practically any expense thrown at the problem.[153] A leading periodical reported in 2015[154] that newly approved cancer drugs can cost from $10,000 to $30,000 per month, up from an average of $4,500 per month a decade ago. Insurance, given that you have it, typically covers 70-80% of the cost, leaving the patient responsible for anywhere from $2,000 to $9,000 per month, on top of their insurance premiums and general living expenses.

Clearly, all of this is acceptable only if this is the best we can expect. How though can anyone settle for that grim prognosis without a solid understanding what causes cancer? Surely that is a gaping hole in the cancer story. How can any cancer patient trust their treatment given that it stems from such uncertainty? Is anyone really surprised that the cost of grasping for straws in such darkness threatens to exceed our means?

Alternative medicine appears to play a complementary role in cancer treatment, strengthening the rest of the body in the hope Nature will prevail in favor of the patient. It too lacks a concise explanation for the cause of cancer, often echoing the mainstream argument that Nature has failed, or that the body has been poisoned. In its defense, it is widely available, and its remedies are typically far less expensive, as well as far kinder to the flesh, than the mainstream solution. Those facts coupled with consistently positive results should have tipped the balance in its favor, becoming the favorite of customers and insurance companies alike. It has not, and I can only conclude that results (or possible legal suppression) are the culprit.

Cancer

That leaves GNM, which offers an elegantly rational explanation of what cancer is, why it occurs, and decidedly optimistic prognoses. Treatment is typically the least expensive of all the solutions, as medicine intended to halt or destroy the cancer cells is understood as at best unnecessary, and surgical intervention is indicated only in emergency situations (blockages, etc.) For all of this, it is outlawed in its country of origin, Germany, and its discoverer, Dr. Hamer, was jailed and hounded into exile upon his release from prison. GNM is known only to a relative few 30+ years after its discovery despite what I perceive as a clear need for effective alternatives to the status quo.

In 1997, Dr. Hamer was arrested for giving three people medical advice without a medical license, which he had been stripped of when he refused to renounce GNM. His patient files were confiscated to be used in the trial against him. Per the rules of discovery, the public prosecutor was forced to admit that after five years (so as to compare apples to apples), 6,000 of 6,500 mostly *terminal* cancer patients were still alive, an astounding 92% survival rate.[155] I can understand why the cancer industry fears this man's discoveries. I cannot understand why anyone else would. It is not technically difficult to test, to confirm yes or no, so I can only conclude that it is politically difficult.

A few brave people have tested Dr. Hamer's discoveries.[156] Most of these occurred before Dr. Hamer's legal troubles, and the subsequent threat of jail time that followed, with the notable exception of the Government of Nicaragua, which officially recognized GNM as a medical therapy in 2011.

Central Nervous System

This chapter deals with disorders of the central nervous system (CNS) other than cancer (see *Cancer* chapter).

Multiple sclerosis (MS) is a CNS disease that interferes with communication between the brain and body and within the brain itself.

Parkinson's Disease (PD) is a neurological disorder, characterized by tremors, that is chronic and degenerative.

Amyotrophic lateral sclerosis (ALS) is a 100% fatal degenerative disease of the nerve cells in the brain and spinal cord.

Organizations

The largest medical charity focusing on multiple sclerosis was founded in 1946.[157] Their mission for these past 71 years has been to rid the world of MS and to heal those currently stricken by the disease. They are organized into three home offices and 71 local offices throughout the United States. Their combined income for 2015 was $214,387,285.[158]

The preeminent medical charity for Parkinson's disease was founded in 2000.[159] They too are dedicated to wiping out their target disease through research and to improving the lives of those afflicted by it. They operate in Canada and the United States of America. Their revenue for 2015 was $99,910,394.[160]

Another large health charity focusing on ALS has been in operation for 32 years, having been founded in 1985.[161] It is their mission to serve, act as advocates for, and to empower victims of ALS so that they may lead full lives, while funding research for treatments and eventually a cure. There are 40 local chapters throughout the United States, as well as a national office. Their total combined revenue for the year ending Jan 31, 2016, was $68,710,377.[162]

The US federal government also funds research into CNS disorders. Their funding, again (my apologies for sounding like a broken record), dwarfs private contributions (see *Appendix*). As usual, all of these efforts focus mainly on allopathic protocols.

Mainstream Theory

Allopathic approaches to disorders of the CNS center on disease management.

Mainstream medicine acknowledges that they do not understand the cause of MS, and that management of the disease is their only recourse, ideally from the very first symptoms. It seems that this paradigm is at a loss how to return a patient with this illness to health, and at this time, can only prescribe treatments that target symptoms, and addresses peripheral complications such as safety (due to impaired motor function) and emotional strength (due to often bleak prognoses). Typical of allopathic research, progress has been made in identifying just what in the CNS is being compromised[163] to cause the symptoms indicating MS. Degradation in nerve sheathing called myelin as well as

Healthcare

the type of (immune) cells that cause the degradation, have been discovered. Some of the receptors on the cells responsible for this apparent attack have also been identified. This paves the way for a drug designed to block those receptors in the hope of stopping the disease. The question of why this is happening remains unanswered, as does the inevitable question of what side effects one can expect by blocking those receptors. Currently, allopathic treatment of MS includes an extensive range of pharmaceuticals that primarily manage symptoms.[164]

Allopathy offers medications and surgery as palliatives for Parkinson's disease (PD), as the cause remains unknown and there is still no cure.[165] Again, I see the same frustration and grim prognosis as with MS. I can also recognize that progress has been made in identifying the culprits in Parkinson's: cell death of neurons in a part of the brain called the substantia nigra, negatively affecting dopamine production. Thus pharmaceutical efforts are targeted in large part at drugs that replace or mimic dopamine.[166]

Finally, mainstream medicine[167] admits that the cause of ALS remains unknown. As before, researchers have discovered that it is the neurons, both upper (brain) and lower (spinal cord), responsible for voluntary muscle movements that gradually degenerate and die in this disease, most often culminating in respiratory failure in the patient. Which cells die has been determined; why they die has not. Treatment is palliative, seeking to delay or reduce symptoms and techniques to deal with the problems that arise from decreased motor activity. The website www.healingals.org is a hub for anecdotal evidence that ALS need not be a death sentence.

It seems the allopathic approach to CNS disorders has not been very successful in eradicating or even checking these diseases. The passion of the doctors and their patients in finding a cure is not in question. As these conditions tend to be progressively debilitating and often, eventually fatal, there is an understandable extreme urgency directed at research, which unfortunately proceeds at full speed without the guidance of cause. Regrettably, the pace at which you careen down a dead end road is only relevant if you intend to change course once you realize you are on a path that leads nowhere. Is allopathy capable of that realization?

Maverick Theory

The three diseases I outline in this chapter all affect motion. That is, they all affect the muscles we use to move. GNM refers to DHS's of this type as motor conflicts, which are a type of self-devaluation conflict.

Motor conflicts are related to the *play-dead* reflexes found in some animals. Simulated death is usually a sudden onset reaction in the wild, seemingly intended to fool a predator into thinking their trapped prey has already died. Why this stops a predator is unknown and irrelevant. It works; it is an effective survival strategy. There are not many parallel circumstances in the modern human experience, so it is difficult to recreate playing dead in humans anecdotally. Certainly, we experience feeling trapped, not being able to move (literally or figuratively), being unable to advance one's position at work, being unable to get out from under relationships, etc. When these conflicts afflict the leg muscles, it has to do with locomotion – being stuck, not being able to run away, sidestep, keep up, follow, etc. When they affect the arms, it has to do with not being able to fight, or embrace, or push away. When they affect the hands, it has to do with not being able to hold or grab something or someone. Conflicts of the facial muscles can involve any of the aspects of *losing face*. A DHS of this type is controlled by the new-brain, indicating initial cell loss (e.g. myelin nerve sheathing), followed by cell gain upon conflict resolution.

GNM views MS as a hanging-active conflict of this nature. The initial shock affects the muscles but is not resolved, so that further cell loss is experienced. If this loss becomes apparent to the patient, noticeably affecting movement, panic may ensue, and another conflict of being unable to escape can be perceived, all before the initial conflict is resolved. A poor prognosis from a medical professional adds to the downward spiral as visions of being wheelchair-bound only further the feeling of being stuck, not being able to move or escape.

When an animal plays dead, if the predator loses interest in the animal and leaves the scene, their conflict is over, and their brains reverse what was done during the crisis. The first outward signs[168] of this are normal breathing, followed by somewhat violent limb twitching, as the animal regains their normal state. This twitching is akin to a seizure, indicative of the healing phase entering the EC state.

This twitching in humans can be indicative of Parkinson's disease. GNM views PD as a hanging-healing of this type of DHS. Unlike MS, the conflict has been resolved, but the tremors that present in the epileptoid crisis (EC) reinforce and deepen the motor conflict. Rather than understanding that the tremors are a temporary healing sign, the patient feels stuck in a body that no longer responds as they wish, and by not understanding what is happening physiologically, are repeatedly relapsed into shock, deepening their particular downward spiral. All resolved SBSs encounter an EC. Some, like PD, are difficult if not impossible to overcome due to ignorance and depth of conflict repetition. Others, as I will show in the next chapter, can be fatal.

Central Nervous System

ALS is another motor conflict that outwardly manifests very similar to MS. Guillain-Barré syndrome (GBS) is another. Mainstream medicine has identified which nerves are compromised in each of these diseases and differentiates based on these discoveries. To GNM, they are just different manifestations of a motor conflict. The *cure* is similar for all, which begins, as do all successful GNM treatments, with a thorough, conscious understanding of cause in the mind of the patient.

Audit

This particular category of conditions suffers from monumentally dismal prognoses from most medical paradigms. In these, ALS is a death sentence, MS & PD are lifelong crippling afflictions that steadily grow worse, and GBS is a roll-the-dice proposition if you will ever fully recover. Cure is never mentioned in connection with these ailments, only treatment. There seems to be nowhere to go but up.

With federal commitment alone pushing nearly $2 billion annually, there is apparently political interest. To date, however, funding has not resulted in much hope, which is not very surprising, given the level of ignorance as to cause. The mainstream knows more today than yesterday of what is happening at the nerve level, as is typical of allopathy, but silence as to why is mostly all that greets patients.

GNM proposes a cause, a reason for the muscle weakness. It also shows how to return to health, although due to the hanging, repetitive, nature of the cause of these conditions, this return becomes more difficult with time. It does, however, offer real hope for a future free from these diseases. Education is the key. Knowledge of the nature of this DHS, and the physiological symptoms to expect during the course of the SBS, are essential in allowing these conflicts to heal.

Heart

This chapter deals with disorders of the heart and coronary veins and arteries other than cancer (see *Cancer* chapter).

Atherosclerosis is a narrowing of the coronary arteries that supply heart with blood flow, due to a buildup of plaque (fat, cholesterol, etc.)

Heart attack (myocardial infarction) occurs when blood flow to the heart is severely restricted or even cut off.

Cardiac arrest is a condition wherein parts of the heart beat erratically, and blood flow ceases.

Cardiomyopathy is a chronic disease of the heart muscle.

High blood pressure refers to the force of the blood flowing through your blood vessels. If it is consistently too high, it can contribute to stroke and heart attack.

Organizations

The preeminent medical charity for heart conditions (and stroke) was founded in 1926.[169] For more than 90 years, they have been dedicated to improving heart health. Their recent campaign sets a goal for the year 2020, to improve the cardiovascular health of all Americans by 20 percent while reducing deaths from diseases of the heart (and stroke) by

20 percent.[170] They are highly organized, with 146 local offices throughout the United States. Their revenue for 2016 was $911.9 million,[171] the bulk of which is covered by private donations.

The US federal government, funds heart disease research to the tune of roughly $4 billion per year (see *Appendix*), a hefty sum, but justified by diseases of the heart taking the lives of approximately 630,000 people in the USA each year. That tops the leading cause-of-death list for the United States.

Mainstream Theory

As I have stated earlier, there are many opinions about what causes disease. Schools of thought differ, as do doctors within a school of thought.

Conventional medical wisdom implicates cholesterol in heart disease. Two types are identified: HDL (the good cholesterol), and LDL (the bad cholesterol). The claim is essentially: too much bad + too little good = eventual clogged arteries,[172] which can lead to a heart attack or stroke, as clots form around broken plaque, blocking blood flow, resulting in heart muscle necrosis. In truth, HDL and LDL are types of lipoproteins[173] which surround cholesterol and enable its transport in blood. The LDL shuttles cholesterol from the liver to cells, while the HDL returns unused cholesterol to the liver. Why one is bad while the other is good is difficult to comprehend; they are both necessary, as is the cholesterol they carry. Allopathy acknowledges that the liver produces all the cholesterol the body needs (to build cells), but maintains that certain foods (saturated and trans fats) in our diet cause the liver to produce an excess of cholesterol, which can lead to the problems mentioned above. I have not been able to ascertain just how

Healthcare

these dietary fats cause the liver to overproduce cholesterol. Perhaps this silence is explained[174] by an average exposure of only 24 (a low of 2, to a high of 70) contact hours (not semester hours, but actual teaching hours) of nutrition instruction over the course of a typical accredited medical degree of approximately 3000 contact hours.

The only person ever to win two unshared Noble prizes was Linus Pauling (Chemistry 1951, Peace 1962). Like allopathic medical doctors, he too saw cholesterol buildup in arteries. That the plaque is there is a fact; why it is there is theory. The mainstream, as mentioned above, endorses a diet based theory. Dr. Pauling agreed with the diet angle, but suggested another reason for the buildup – chronic vitamin C deficiency.[175]

The human liver, unlike that in many mammals, apparently lacks the enzyme L-gulonolactone oxidase (GULO) to convert glucose to vitamin C.[176] This is a potential health issue as vitamin C is essential for the production of collagen, and relatively large amounts of collagen are required to maintain blood vessels, bones, skin, tendons, ligaments, teeth, and organs. Without it, we basically fall apart. Chronic vitamin C deficiency has a name – scurvy. Dr. Pauling proposed that arterial cholesterol buildup was being used by the body as a patch to repair blood vessels rendered structurally unsound by a chronic lack of vitamin C. He saw it as a bad/worse choice for the brain. Either risk heart attack and stroke from blood clots formed around the plaque, or bleed to death internally from a ruptured blood vessel. The arteries and veins near the heart are subject to the most mechanical stress due to its pumping action and are therefore most in need of the maintenance vitamin C enables. If this theory is correct, surgically scraping away the cholesterol removes the patch, re-exposing the weakened blood vessels to the pressures from the heart, exactly what your brain was trying to avoid by building the patch in the first place. Bypassing the damaged vessels with blood vessels lifted from your leg (bypass surgery) does nothing to address the cause. Was Dr. Pauling more correct than the establishment? Let us apply Occam's razor. Eat more Vitamin C (lots of raw fruits and vegetables) and monitor the heart blood vessels closely, or assume Nature has once again lost her mind, and risk open heart surgery? Surgery may be necessary, as the patient may find themselves in an emergency situation, but I wonder how many such patients are chronically deficient in Vitamin C?

Cardiac arrest is a condition wherein the electrical signals from the brain controlling the beating of your heart are somehow altered, effectively interrupting the pumping action, and killing you unless the electrical signal can be reset. Watch enough police or hospital TV shows, and you can't help but understand how that is accomplished, cardio pulmonary resuscitation (CPR) and cardioversion, accompanied by the familiar *clear* warning. There is also a chemical (pharmaceutical) cardioversion.

What does the mainstream have to say about why the electrical signals malfunction?[177]

- **Heart muscle scarring.** Let's try to get at the root cause, which would rule out a previous heart attack.
- **Cardiomyopathy.** Typically caused by high blood pressure or valvular heart disease. What causes high blood pressure? Conventional wisdom splinters the answer into many risk factors, while other allopathic health resources are more forthcoming in stating that the causes of high blood pressure are unknown.[178] What causes valvular heart disease? According to medical authorities,[179] mostly high blood pressure, heart failure, atherosclerosis, heart attack, rheumatic

123

fever (0.3% of people with strep throat). Is this not circular reasoning?
- **Pharmaceuticals.** The medicine intended to prevent cardiac arrest can apparently cause cardiac arrest! That's not good.
- **Electrical problems.** Allopaths suspect Wolff-Parkinson-White syndrome. Well, what causes that? An organization dedicated to rare illnesses[180] states that WPW occurs randomly for no apparent reason. In other words: they don't know. Long QT syndrome is also indicated and blamed on genetics. Both of these syndromes are listed as rare disorders.
- **Irregular blood vessels.** These are birth defects, apparently responsible for some of the cardiac arrests in athletes, where athletic stress breaks a vital body part. These are very rare.
- **Illegal drugs.** Besides the claim being quite vague, this reason is seemingly also rare.

So it appears that the most significant threats of cardiac arrest are: having a weak or damaged heart, high blood pressure, and heart medication. At any rate, prompt attention is essential to survival, as the chance of death increases 10% for every minute delay, essentially summoning the Grim Reaper if ten minutes are allowed to pass without medical intervention.

A noninvasive, FDA approved procedure called enhanced external counterpulsation[181] (EECP) uses compression synchronized to your heartbeat to relieve symptoms of ischemic heart diseases. It is typically used when surgery is not an option.

Alternative Theory

In TCM, every organ is seen to have responsibilities, beyond the physical. Each is regarded as having a soul attribute. The heart is the ruler of the other organs in this regard, being endowed with Shen, which coordinates this spiritual sense. TCM recognizes the following heart patterns: Chi Deficiency, Yang Deficiency, Blood deficiency, Yin Deficiency, Fire Blazing, Blood Stagnation. Acupuncture with and without moxa (burning herb) is indicated to rebalance chi.

Ayurveda attributes heart disease largely to stress and elevated blood pressure and addresses those issues with meditation, herbs, and diet.

One line of thinking relates clogged arteries with heavy metal poisoning and recommends (since 1955) chelation therapy[182] as an aid in returning the blood vessels supplying the heart to a healthier state.

Stress reduction, diet (including supplements, in particular, coenzyme Q10) and exercise round out the bulk of preventive strategies used by the alternative health community. Numerous alternative paradigms employ these tactics when treating heart disease.

Maverick Theory

As stated previously, Dr. Hamer has meticulously mapped organs with control relays in the brain. Each relay will react to different DHSs. The human heart is associated with several different brain relays, and as such, is susceptible to many different conflict shocks.

Healthcare

The right and left ventricles are responsible for carrying blood out of the heart. They consist of 90% striated muscle, and 10% smooth muscle.

The striated muscle, responsible for contraction, is controlled by the motor cortex. This myocardial tissue is affected by relationship conflicts, specifically such conflicts relating to feeling completely overwhelmed, not by work, but by other people. During the first phase of an SBS (CA), this muscle experiences necrosis, which is reversed during the second phase (PCL) (can be diagnosed as myocardial sarcoma — if inflamed, myocarditis), revealing the biological purpose behind the SBS, which is a stronger myocardium. Laterality applies (left or right handed – see *The Maverick Solution* chapter), so the symptom, which presents during the epileptoid crisis (EC), is either a left or a right myocardial infarct, or heart attack. This crisis is triggered in the heart rhythm center of the brain. Dr. Hamer observed that the EC will occur within 48 hours of conflict resolution, and its intensity is proportional to the intensity and duration of the CA phase. Downgrading a conflict will lessen the intensity, but resolving the conflict will lead to the EC, which is often a moment of truth. If the patient endured the conflict for too long a time, or the conflict was too intense, the EC will most likely prove fatal. Necrosis during the CA phase can lead to a noticeable weakening of affected ventricle, leading to a diagnosis of congestive heart failure.

The smooth muscle, responsible for tissue nutrition, is controlled by the cerebral medulla. It is affected by a conflict of not being able to transport sufficient amounts of blood. The EC for this SBS is rarely noticed.

The left and right atria are responsible for carrying blood into the heart. They consist of smooth muscle and are controlled by the midbrain. This myocardial tissue is affected by conflicts related to not being able to move enough blood (peristalsis). Dr. Hamer identified a poor medical diagnosis as a significant source of this conflict. Cell gain during CA phase is not reversed during PCL phase, a characteristic shared with all midbrain SBSs. Symptoms are again present in the EC, presenting as a type of colic, as expected from the healing phase of peristaltic tissue.

The pericardium is a layered membrane that protects the heart. It reacts to attacks against the heart by thickening (cell growth). These attacks can be physical (localized to the area of the heart), or abstract, for example in the form of an unfavorable diagnosis (you have a heart condition), or sharp insults (cut to the heart). Sufficient cell growth here can be diagnosed by mainstream medicine as a pericardial mesothelioma (a heart tumor that grows in a flat plane). Pericardial effusion (fluid buildup) occurs during PCL (healing) phase, which applies pressure to the heart muscle and can be amplified to dangerous levels by kidney collecting tubule syndrome (KCTS). Pressure applied to the heart in this manner due to acutely elevated levels of fluid in the healing pericardium can result in cardiac arrest and is known as cardiac tamponade.

Coronary arteries and veins feed the heart muscle and are affected by territorial-loss conflicts in males (or postmenopausal females) or sexual conflicts in menstrual age females (distress concerning sexuality – abuse, harassment, rejection, unexpected separation or loss). During CA phase, the internal cells of these blood vessels ulcerate, resulting in a larger area for blood to flow and often, a diagnosis of angina pectoris. Cholesterol is used to restore the ulcerated lining during the healing phase (PCL). A blood test during this time will most likely indicate an elevated cholesterol level. A hanging-healing can result in arteriosclerosis, as more and more cholesterol is employed in the repair. A KCTS can amplify the swelling that marks the healing phase to the point of blocking the blood vessel, but the real danger in conflicts affecting these blood vessels, comes in the EC, just like most heart-related SBSs. All cellular repair happens in a fluid medium, and the brain is no exception. During the EC, which will occur 2-6 weeks after conflict resolution (depending on conflict intensity and duration), this fluid is expelled, resulting in pressure on the affected brain relays. This pressure can disturb the electrical connection to the corresponding organ, and in the case of the heart, even result in cardiac arrest. In the coronary veins, the EC will involve the striated musculature of the vein, resulting in cramping. During this physical stress, plaque may be dislodged, and travel to the lungs, where it may cause a pulmonary embolism (blockage of a lung artery).

How does GNM challenge Dr. Pauling's observations of scurvy and arterial damage? GNM claims that cholesterol is being used to repair the blood vessel (cholesterol is a significant membrane constituent of animal cells).[183] Dr. Pauling claimed that cholesterol is used as a temporary patch. GNM claims that blood vessels are ulcerated for temporary biological advantage, just as other cells in the body are, requiring restoration, and therefore cholesterol, after conflict resolution. Dr. Pauling claimed that blood vessels (and presumably other tissue), are structurally compromised by vitamin C deficiency and that restoring vitamin C levels facilitates cell repair, through cholesterol and collagen. I can see how both of these scenarios are possible, as they do not contradict one another. They might even occur simultaneously. One involves (mal)nutrition, the other, a biologically meaningful response to conflict shock.

Audit

Along with Occam's razor seeming to favor Dr. Pauling's vitamin C therapy over non-emergency open heart surgery, that solution has the added benefit of being by comparison, practically free. GNM is also almost free in contrast, while offering a much higher degree of diagnostic detail. Actual monitoring (CT scan, etc.) is however not free.

Ultimately, the main reason I can see that most people die of heart issues has to do with (the lack of) time, with the sudden and catastrophic nature of the complications, as well as the relative ignorance on the part of the patients of the extent of their problem, as the mainstream understanding of cause seems to me vague at best. If help arrives immediately, you stand some chance of living through these complications, if it takes more than 10 minutes, chances are, you're probably dead. This rules out using GNM or vitamin C therapy for emergency situations. They both require an understanding of what is happening, and the time to address the cause, and effect repairs.

This fact (time) forces every heart ailment survival strategy into the realm of prevention. For me, there are far too many holes in the allopathic understanding of heart disease for my comfort, and far too many failures (deaths) because of this issue for me to blindly embrace the mainstream suggestions for prevention. GNM is again unique in that it predicts when complications will occur (during the EC, which occurs midway through PCL [SBS phase 2], which is as long in duration as CA [SBS phase 1]), allowing for at least some preparation. It also is the only paradigm that offers an active response to prevention. By that, I mean that if GNM is correct, you stand some chance of minimizing potential attacks through the recognition of cause. With others, you are hoping or praying your preventive measures will work.

The nature of a heart attack will, regardless of which medical strategy you embrace, land you in the emergency room should such a crisis occur. Once your heart has stopped, anyplace other than an ER, or its extension, an ambulance, is of little help.

Kidneys and Bladder

This chapter deals with disorders of the kidneys and bladder other than cancer (see *Cancer* chapter).

Chronic kidney disease (CKD) is defined as kidneys that are not filtering as they should. In other words, they are underperforming.

Diseases of the bladder include cystitis, which is an inflammation.

Organizations

The largest medical charity for kidney health was founded in 1950 to support kidney patients and their families. Today, 67 year later, it is organized into 17 local chapters across the USA. Revenue for 2017 was $39,483,934.[184]

US federal commitment through the National Institutes for Health is predictably larger, by more than an order of magnitude (see *Appendix*).

Mainstream Theory

Allopathy identifies five stages of kidney disease.[185] The fifth, or final stage is when the patient requires a kidney transplant or dialysis to live. Allopathic kidney treatment rests on a foundation of two measurements: ACR, or albumin to creatinine ratio and GFR, or glomerular filtration rate. ACR measures elevated proteins in urine. GFR measures the flow rate of filtered fluid through the kidney in milliliters per minute. Allopaths assign a stage number based on GFR. This number is used in determining which treatments are indicated.

Stage	Description	GFR
1	Kidney damage with normal kidney function	>90
2	Kidney damage with mild loss of kidney function	60-89
3a	Mild to moderate loss of kidney function	44-59
3b	Moderate to severe loss of kidney function	30-44
4	Severe loss of kidney function	15-39
5	Kidney failure	<15

Mainstream medical kidney strategy involves adjustments to diet and medication to treat the symptoms associated with CKD as allopaths have noticed a correlation between CKD and diabetes and high blood pressure. The aim is to slow the disease, as allopaths concede they have no cure.[186]

Maverick Theory

Water is an essential resource for life. A human adult can live for months without food but will perish in under a week without water. A person has some voluntary control over conserving the nutrients and energy they have consumed in the form of food. Physical exertion will consume the food faster than sitting still, doing nothing. Water, on the other hand, is exhaled (as vapor) with every breath, and sweat is necessary to cool the skin during hot weather. These bodily functions are not under conscious control. The kidneys, or more specifically, the kidney-collecting-tubules (KCT), are responsible for collecting urine

Healthcare

produced in the kidney parenchyma (up to 2 liters per day), and moving it out of the body.

GNM relies heavily on embryology and historical evolution to understand how the brain and body react to events. The kidneys, in their role of water processor, appear to have been endowed with the ability to regulate the amount of water released based on perceived threats. Conflicts of abandonment (existence, hospitalization, refugee, isolation) can affect the kidneys, which may respond by severely restricting the amount of water processed out of the body. Remember that all conflict shocks are subjective. Just because someone is hospitalized, or isolated, or abandoned does not mean that they will experience a DHS. When any SBS (2-phase reaction to DHS) is in the healing phase (PCL), and a conflict shock of the sort mentioned above does occur, the patient will experience what Dr. Hamer has called kidney collecting tubule syndrome (KCTS), or simply "the syndrome"

This SBS retains water throughout the body, as the collecting tubules in effect, clam up. This results in an amplification of the healing symptoms of the first SBS. Pain, inflammation, and swelling are all exaggerated because of the excess water. The syndrome can radically complicate any healing process, so the GNM strategy is to resolve a KCT DHS as soon as possible so that this symptom amplification will subside. This understanding is also unique to GNM as far as I can tell. It was Dr. Hamer's opinion that KCTS was our leading cause of death.

Kidneys are an embryologically complex organ. By that I mean that control of the kidneys occurs in several locations within the brain, spanning endoderm to ectoderm. According to Dr. Hamer, the kidney collecting tubules (affected by conflicts of being alone) and the adrenal medulla (affected by conflicts involving unbearably intense stress) are controlled by the brainstem. The conflict-active (CA) period is marked by cell proliferation, which if prolonged can result in visible tumors: adrenal cancer (pheochromocytoma) in the adrenal medulla, and renal cell carcinoma in the KCT.

The adrenal cortex (affected by conflicts of wrong choice), and kidney parenchyma (affected by conflicts related to water or fluid), are controlled by the cerebral medulla. A CA period here is marked by necrosis, which if prolonged can result in Addison's disease in the adrenal cortex, and hypertension (high blood pressure) in the kidney parenchyma (followed by kidney cysts [Wilms' tumor] in the PCL).

The cerebrum controls the renal pelvis and ureters (both affected by territorial marking conflicts). Epithelial ulcers (cell loss) mark the CA period, followed by kidney colic (kidney gravel or stones can form due to a hanging-healing) in the PCL.

The bladder is used in the animal kingdom to hold enough urine to mark a territory effectively. A common biological response to boundary conflicts is to enable more urine flow to better mark the boundary. This is accomplished via ulceration of the urethra to widen the urine channel. Cell necrosis during this phase is accompanied by numbness, which allows urine flow without pain. The healing phase reverses this process, and urine flow will irritate new cell/nerve connections, resulting in a burning sensation and possibly blood. If bacteria, which GNM proposes are there to assist in repairs, are present in the PCL phase, an examination by a mainstream doctor would most likely yield a diagnosis of a urinary tract or bladder infection (aka cystitis).

Bedwetting is a not uncommon childhood experience. It too is a symptom of a marking conflict (bullying, siblings not respecting personal space, etc.). The wetting incident(s) occur during the EC phase, in the middle of PCL, a vagotonic (resting, sleep) state.

Healthcare

Audit

Medicare alone shells out $34 billion per year for dialysis.[187] At a cost of roughly $88,000 per patient per year, including emergency room visits and hospitalization, this strategy, for an estimated 650,000 US citizens and rising, appears to me to be unsustainable.

The alternative to end stage renal failure (ESRF), for which dialysis is the current mainstream go-to treatment, is kidney transplant. The costs of this option are $32,000 for the transplant surgery and $25,000 per year for maintenance. In 2014, there were only 17,000 donor kidneys available for transplant.[188]

To my thinking, that is a lot of money for a maintenance plan. Nowhere in these two strategies is a *cure*. Nowhere is there a promise of returning to a normal life. If you transplant a kidney and do not address why the kidney failed, how long will it be before you land back on that donor waiting list? Saying that high blood pressure and diabetes are the cause of kidney failure is to push the reason onto two other conditions for which mainstream medicine is seemingly also unsure as to cause. Is this really our best and final foot forward?

GNM presents a clear path forward for kidney disease. It identifies cause and clues to conflict resolution. As the inevitable outcome of the mainstream solution seems to be ESRF, why are alternative theories being ignored? If for nothing more than financial reasons, why aren't insurance companies exploring this space with patients? Surely many patients are none too keen about the gloomy mainstream prognosis of renal failure. Dr. Hamer estimated that "In GNM, kidney transplants become unnecessary in about 90% of cases, provided the underlying existence conflict can be resolved".[189] Why is this being ignored?

Liver and Gallbladder

This chapter deals with disorders of the liver and gallbladder other than cancer (see *Cancer* chapter).

Hepatitis is an inflammation that causes the liver to swell.

Cirrhosis is scarring of the liver.

Organizations

The largest medical charity for liver health was founded in 1976. For 41 years it has sought to prevent, treat, and eventually cure diseases of the liver, by facilitating support, promoting education and funding research. Today, it is organized into 24 local offices across the USA. Revenue for 2017 was $9,647,270.[190]

Federal spending on diseases of the liver and gallbladder are considerably higher, approaching $1 billion per year (see *Appendix*). This outlay is commensurate with alcohol popularity, which saw more than half of the population admitting to imbibing in the last month, and more than a quarter of the population admitting to binge drinking in that same span.[191] The liver processes alcohol, so naturally, alcohol abuse burdens the liver, which may lead to liver health issues.

Mainstream Theory

Allopathy claims to have identified up to 6 different strains of virus that primarily attack the liver. They are hepatitis A, B, C, D, E and G viruses (HAV, HBV, HCV, etc.). Types A, B and C are supposedly the most common. All types are implicated in acute hepatitis, whereas only types B and C are implicated in chronic hepatitis.

Mainstream medicine's approach to treatment is based on which strain of hepatitis virus is involved. The medical mainstream informs us that hepatitis-A is rarely treated medically, as it usually clears up within six months.[192] The same approach is also taken with adults diagnosed with acute hepatitis B, as most recover fully without medication. An arsenal of antiviral drugs are used to treat chronic cases (5%), often the same drugs employed to treat HIV.[193] Acute hepatitis C is largely asymptomatic and is therefore rarely treated,[194] although pharmaceuticals do exist to manage hepatitis C symptoms.

Since the large majority of acute hepatitis cases are left untreated, why is so much effort expended on diagnosis (especially A & B)? Is it because mainstream therapies & theory too often fail to prevent cases from becoming chronic? Vaccines are the allopathic go-to prophylactic for hepatitis. They are reportedly made from attenuated viruses, which logically presupposes that a virus has been isolated to attenuate. This strategy explicitly relies on the ability not only to identify hepatitis virus but further, the particular type of hepatitis virus. How is that done?

The symptoms of acute hepatitis include dark-colored urine, light-colored stool, jaundice, and fatigue. Chronic hepatitis seems to lack distinct symptoms. These are the observed facts. Why this happens is where theory and axiom come into play. Pasteurian Germ Theory proposes that microbes are responsible for infections. Allopathy has adopted Germ Theory as axiom, that is, a proposition accepted as fact. Hepatitis is an inflamed liver, indicating infection. It is only natural then that allopaths suspect a responsible microbe in such cases. In many persons exhibiting hepatitis symptoms, bacteria, toxins, parasites, etc. are ruled out. Enter the virus responsible for hepatitis. With an optical microscope, a trained person can quickly identify bacteria. The same cannot be said for viruses, as they are apparently too small.

How then did researchers initially hunt for this never-before-seen hepatitis virus? Well, it appears to me that first you must assume they exist. Immunology is an outgrowth of Germ Theory. It attempts to explain how the body defends against invading microbes. In 1900, Paul Ehrlich proposed the Side Chain Theory[195] whereby a host-produced antibody molecule was able to bind to receptors on the surface of a microbe. In general terms, this model is still apparently viable today. As late as 1970, nobody had seen, isolated or concentrated this suspected virus thought to be responsible for hepatitis-A. Then in 1971, researchers published papers describing a process called the enzyme-linked immunosorbent assay (ELISA).[196] ELISA was designed to signal antibodies binding to antigens by observing color changes in test material. It would prove invaluable in the quest to identify viruses.

HAV was first positively identified in 1973.[197] The report indicates that HAV antibodies were used to coat the virus so that it could be visualized with an electron microscope. How HAV antibodies were identified without an isolated HAV is not specified, resulting, in my opinion, in a catch-22 that permeates viral investigation.

A blood sample is drawn from a patient showing symptoms of liver disease and therefore suspected of hosting a hepatitis virus. Since the hepatitis virus is assumed to be present, it is logical to assume that some hepatitis antibodies are also present, at least in patients with working immune systems. If ELISA is seeded with hepatitis antibodies, they will bind to the unbound hepatitis viruses in the blood sample. If ELISA is seeded with hepatitis virus, they will bind to the unbound hepatitis antibodies in the blood sample. Either way, after some enzyme chemistry, a color change should be observed indicating the presence of these bonds.

At this point, to my layman's understanding, ELISA is making sense. However, what I'm having trouble with, is understanding how the seed material, necessary for ELISA to do its thing, is procured. If you are testing blood for the presence of HAV, you need mostly pure HAV antibodies. Likewise, if you are testing for HAV antibodies, you need mostly pure HAV. If the seed is not pure, how will you know what is binding to what? Science calls unknowns such as these confounding variables, and strongly encourages avoidance.

Assuming that blood from a patient with suspected hepatitis has more HAV than HAV antibodies, the first test should focus on preparing an antibody seed. So, how are antibodies isolated? How do you get a pure amount? A common method involves the preparation of antigen samples that are then injected into animals, whose immune systems then supposedly react to the presence of these antigens and produce high levels of antibodies, which are then recovered from the animal.[198] To elaborate:

1. A large load of unbound hepatitis virus (antigen) is assumed to be present in blood collected from a person suffering from what has been diagnosed as hepatitis.
2. This blood is then prepared, presumably to isolate the virus. There are several ways to accomplish this. A relatively crude way is by size-exclusion through filtration. How small should this filter be if you've not yet isolated and thus measured the

Liver And Gallbladder

virus? What else passes through that filter? A specific way is by antibody affinity, a technique that assumes a pure antibody sample, which for HAV in 1970 was putting the cart before the horse. Logically, it produces bound/neutralized viruses.

3. This sample is then injected into an animal host. It is assumed to be mostly the target virus, though that is a function of isolation method.
4. Time is allowed to lapse, during which it is assumed that the animal host immune system is reacting to the suspected virus and producing many more antibodies than there are viruses, so that there will be unbound antibodies to collect. Why the host should produce this excess is unspecified. That a species other than human is used for incubation, is of no apparent concern; why this should be is a complete mystery to me.
5. Then antibodies, along with who knows what else (at least some neutralized viruses, presumably), are collected from the unwitting virus incubator in the form of blood samples, which are then subjected to a similar isolation method, presumably to isolate the unbound antibodies.
6. This soup of tiny bits is declared to be a specific antibody concentrate and then used as an ELISA seed.

Nowhere is the virus actually isolated, nowhere is it seen. It is merely assumed to be present, as Germ Theory predicts. The non-human host incubator is assumed to react to the injection of this isolate by creating a surplus of human compatible HAV antibodies. The potential presence of confounding variables is ignored, as if a pure virus was injected into the incubator, which has not been established. How any tiny bits from the animal host that manage to slip through the second isolation affect fresh human blood samples is unknowable (since they are unidentified), and also seemingly ignored. Nowhere is the antibody actually isolated. It is merely assumed to be present as immunology predicts. How can this be? Does this house of cards form the general basis for allopathic hepatitis virus testing? Hint: it appears to have formed, at least initially, the basis for all of allopathic virus testing! Invalidate one assumption, and this whole process collapses. Perhaps if I look into how viruses are isolated, I will find an easier to understand solution, one that requires embracing fewer assumptions on faith.

How are viruses isolated? How do you get a pure amount? More to the point, how were viruses isolated in the early 1970s when HAV was first identified? Perhaps HBV vaccine production[199] will offer clues, as every HAV vaccine source I could find assumed an isolated HAV: "isolation of genome from virus is the first step". Already, we have a problem. This first step also assumes we have an isolated virus. How did that happen? Using procedures similar to those outlined above? Those are unfortunately burdened by the hefty stack of questionable assumptions previously noted. What am I missing here? Why is this so convoluted? This conundrum mirrors the same problematic assumptions highlighted in the *Virus* chapter regarding measles vaccine.

This exploration is occurring in the *Liver* chapter of this book, but apparently I could just as relevantly placed it anywhere a viral cause for illness is implicated by mainstream medicine. HIV (AIDS), smallpox, polio, measles, HPV, mumps, shingles, herpes, etc. Some of these viruses were *discovered* after HAV, and some before, when the science was presumably less advanced. The pile of assumptions that questions these explanations of cause should give pause to anyone who is simply willing to look. They all share the underlying assumption created by Germ Theory. If this all seems surreal to you, I understand.

I'll move on to cirrhosis, which conventional medicine attributes to other liver diseases, so it's a consequence, not a disease per se, at least not one you can treat. The goal of allopathy in cirrhosis is to stop, or at least minimize, further damage. If liver disease has damaged a liver beyond salvage, then transplant is the last card in the allopath's hand.

One function of the liver is to produce bile, which the gallbladder then stores, only to secrete it into the small intestine later to aid in digesting fats. Gallbladder removal surgery is one of the most common operations with over 700,000 performed yearly in the USA alone. Mainstream medicine's approach to a diseased gallbladder is essentially the same as that for an appendix, removal by surgery. From what I could gather, relatively little (allopathic) effort is expended on understanding gallbladder disease, as one can indeed live without the organ, and barring complications, its removal is considered outpatient surgery.

Alternative medicine has identified ten distinct diseases of the gallbladder,[200] with a list as long as your arm of potential causes.[201] There are more than 30 items on the list. Working your way through it, trying to eliminate all that don't apply to you is going to take a very long time, barring a lucky guess. This, of course, assumes the lists are comprehensive and accurate.

Maverick Theory

The liver is vulnerable to two distinct types of psychic shocks, owing to the nature of the tissues involved. The majority of the liver is endodermal in origin and is therefore subject to morsel conflicts. The rest is ectodermal in origin and thus subject to territorial conflicts.

The functions of the parenchyma or the endodermal liver tissue are many but are ultimately tied to metabolism, of extracting and transforming food into usable nutrients. Thus, a starvation conflict can impact the liver, forming more cells initially (to better utilize all the available nutrients in your food). Should the conflict not resolve for an extended period, a visit to an oncologist could very well confirm liver cancer (see *Cancer* chapter for more details).

The liver bile ducts and the gallbladder are composed of different tissue and are subject to conflict shocks of a different type, namely a territorial-anger conflict, which can result from disputes over money. The ulcerative widening of the bile ducts during the conflict-active (CA) phase of this SBS improves bile flow, resulting in better metabolism, and therefore more energy, to better resolve the conflict. The healing phase (PCL) of this type of conflict shock results in swelling and inflammation and is called hepatitis by mainstream medicine. If during this PCL, an active existence conflict is also present (see KCTS in *Kidneys and Bladder* chapter), this can lead to increased swelling in the bile ducts (hepatomegaly), resulting in an enlarged liver and jaundice (as bile is not able to flow due to duct closure from swelling). In this view, it is not necessary to invent a hypothetical submicroscopic culprit (virus) to blame as cause.

Scarring is a normal consequence of PCL-B, or the second healing phase (after the EC). When this scarring noticeably hinders the flow of bile, mainstream medicine calls this cirrhosis. Such a buildup of scar tissue occurs in the bile ducts as a result of multiple territorial-anger conflicts, or a hanging-healing of such a conflict. This healing phase is also affected by KCTS, resulting in what mainstream medicine refers to as cirrhotic ascites, as water is retained in the abdominal cavity.

The gallbladder is a biological extension of the liver bile ducts, and as such, is also affected by territorial anger conflicts. The PCL phase reverses the cell loss incurred in the CA phase, with accompanying swelling (edema), the magnitude of which is proportional to the duration and intensity of the conflict. A KCTS may also exacerbate the

Liver And Gallbladder

swelling, which can lead to a duct blockage so that bile accumulates. A hanging-healing, where the healing process is interrupted by either tracks or new conflicts, can cause enough bile to accumulate to eventually form gallstones (stones may grow wherever bile accumulates, which includes the liver bile ducts).

Audit

As reported in the press, $9 billion will be spent by Medicare on HCV drugs in 2015.[202] That's just for HCV. They further report that 3 million US citizens are infected with HCV, which allegedly claims more lives in America than AIDS. The same report lists a price tag for these medications of $80,000 to $100,000 per treatment. As acute HCV infection is said to be largely asymptomatic, and therefore mostly untreated, the medication must be intended for sufferers of chronic hepatitis C of which scarring (cirrhosis or fibrosis) is the symptom. This expense does not include the costs of HAV and HBV medicines or vaccines. Nor does it include organ replacement or removal surgeries. The global vaccine (all vaccines) market is estimated to have been $52 billion in 2016.[203] Gallbladder surgery alone can cost upwards of $100,000, though the mean seems more in the $15,000 range. Given 700,000 operations yearly, the cost of this issue alone, assuming the mean price, is roughly $10.5 billion.

That's an awful lot of territorial-anger if GNM is correct. As reason dictates, it should be much cheaper to deal with cause, than to play whack-a-mole with symptoms. Another relatively inexpensive option here comes courtesy of herbalists, who discovered centuries ago that a liver flush[204] can remove stones and chaff en-masse and without pain, thereby preventing the complications and trauma of passing stones normally, and helping to clean and therefore preserve your gallbladder.

Lungs

This chapter deals with disorders of the lungs other than cancer (see *Cancer* chapter).

Influenza (flu) as a highly contagious respiratory illness caused by viruses. Flu can often lead to pneumonia.

Chronic obstructive pulmonary disease (COPD) is defined as a lung disease marked by breathing difficulties. It is also called chronic bronchitis or emphysema.

Cystic fibrosis (CF) is a genetic disease of the lungs. It is characterized by an abundance of thick mucus that progressively limits the ability to breathe.

Organizations

The largest and most well known medical charity dedicated to lung health was founded in 1904, initially to combat tuberculosis.[205] Their stated goal is to save lives by improving lung health. They have funded education, advocacy and research in this pursuit for well over a century. They have a contact in every state in the US, as well as an extensive online presence. Lung issues falling under their umbrella include asthma, COPD, influenza, lung cancer, pneumonia, and smoking. Their revenue for 2015 was $42,840,838.[206]

US Federal funding for lung health issues, as usual, dwarfs private spending (see *Appendix*).

Mainstream Theory

Allopathy regards pneumonia as a respiratory system complication. It is commonly linked with the flu, but also with more than 30 other vectors, in direct violation of Koch's first postulate. Bacteria, viruses, mycoplasmas, fungi, and various chemicals are all implicated in the illness, complicating and obscuring any attempt at a concise understanding of cause. Pneumonia, and its co-conspirator, influenza, are the very definition of a set of symptoms being labeled a disease. Allopathic treatments are palliative, and the common prognosis is that your body will recover in one to three weeks.

Mainstream medicine maintains that there are three known types of influenza viruses, with hundreds, if not thousands, of subtypes and strains. All of which are implicated in causing the flu, a disease primarily affecting the respiratory system, but one that can affect the whole body. Up to 50,000 people die each year in the USA alone of this illness and its complications, though most people recover within a week of symptom onset. Vaccines are the primary flu defense offered by allopathy. According to mainstream authorities, the viral mix varies from year to year, and as such, vaccines are designed for a given mix, in an attempt to cover the strains deemed most likely to cause illness in the coming year. Accounting for all known viral variations is at present impossible. Other treatments are, like those for pneumonia, palliative.

Tuberculosis is one of the top 10 causes of death worldwide. Mainstream medicine defines it as an infectious disease caused by the bacterium *mycobacterium tuberculosis*, and while it typically affects the lungs, it can be found in any organ of the body. I find the allopathic description of tuberculosis[207] puzzling. It maintains that a person with TB infection will be asymptomatic, much like acute hepatitis C. Presumably, this means that such a person tests positive for the bacteria in their blood while showing no signs of the disease. Symptoms of active TB disease include a persistent or bloody cough, fever, loss of appetite, night sweats, weight loss, and fatigue. So it seems that the mere presence of the TB bacteria is insufficient to cause the disease for which it is blamed, a direct violation of Koch's third postulate. The explanation offered by medical authorities is that people with weak immune systems (though not everyone) are in danger of having the TB infection progress to the TB disease. The World Health Organization (WHO) estimates a 10% risk of falling ill with TB for those infected with the bacteria[208], adding that a compromised immune system results in a much higher risk. I find this all very odd. Healthy people riddled with potentially harmful but for some reason latent bacteria, which the immune system largely ignores, as indicated by a lack of typical infection symptoms (fever, sweats, etc.). Ignores, that is, until such time as the immune system weakens, which will somehow trigger an attack by the bacteria. This attack will finally elicit a by now feeble immune response, such that the TB will threaten to overcome the patient without the aid of pharmaceuticals. Perhaps TB bacteria exist for reasons as yet unknown to mainstream medicine.

Allopathy defines asthma as a chronic (often lifelong) disease for which there is no cure. This glum prognosis actually requires a suffix, *using our treatments*, and is again predictable, given their assessment of cause, which is that *nobody understands the exact cause of asthma.*[209] You could convince me that no allopath understands, but such prognoses display an arrogance I already dismissed in an earlier chapter, *The Cure For Disease*. Mainstream treatment of asthma, given the above observations, is unsurprisingly palliative. Rescue inhalers provide emergency relief in the form of albuterol, a muscle relaxer that quickly relaxes bronchial constriction.

Cystic fibrosis is classified by allopathy as a genetic (inherited) disease. Pulmonary infections, and sinus as well as gastrointestinal problems are the hallmarks of this disease. The culprit in this condition is an abnormal version of a protein called cystic fibrosis transmembrane regulator. Why the protein becomes abnormal is presently unclear. Allopathic treatment of this disease consists of medications targeted at thinning mucus or treating infections that result from the mucus, as well as digestive enzymes to supplement the output of the pancreas. Advances in such palliative treatments have raised the life expectancy of CF patients from childhood to nearly 40 years.

The Western world has vilified the smoking of tobacco. The assertion that smoking causes lung cancer is accepted as fact. The reasoning is, that toxins are present in tobacco smoke (clearly this is true: nicotine [toxic, as well as addictive], tar, carbon monoxide, formaldehyde, and ammonia are all present) and that these toxins cause lung cells to mutate. While I can readily agree with the first conclusion (toxins are present, and it is difficult to see how they can be anything but harmful to your health), I am not onboard with the second. Certainly, not everyone who smokes *gets* lung cancer. It has been estimated that fewer than 10% of lifelong smokers will *get* lung cancer.[210] So, why aren't the alveoli of the other 90+% mutating in this toxic fog?

Maverick Theory

Territorial-fear (male), or nest-fear (female), are conflicts associated with bronchial issues. Threats to territory (job, house, etc.) or nest (home, family, etc.) can result in this type of DHS (conflict shock). The

Healthcare

SBS (2-phase response to DHS) that runs in response to such conflicts seeks to ulcerate, and thus, widen the bronchial pathways, allowing for increased oxygen intake. Once the conflict is resolved, the ulcerated cells are replaced in a fluid medium, aided by bacteria. Mainstream medicine labels this condition bronchitis. Should bronchitis be accompanied by the syndrome (KCTS), the diagnosis will be pneumonia. They are the same SBS, according to GNM, differing only in that one is exacerbated by retained water.

The common cold is a disease attributed by mainstream medicine to any one of roughly 100 type of rhinovirus. Like influenza, there are too many continually shifting (evolving?) targets to affect a *cure*. Thankfully, unlike influenza, the disease is usually relatively mild, however inconvenient, so there is no vaccine – yet. The symptoms are similar to influenza, only less severe. GNM distinguishes cold from flu simply by conflict intensity: low intensity = cold, high intensity = flu. The GNM explanation of this melange of symptoms involves the following. Olfactory cells, responsible for our sense of smell, are present in the back of the nasal cavity. A stink conflict will result in the ulceration of those cells (so as not to have to smell the offensive stench), followed, on conflict resolution, by cell regrowth, which occurs in a fluid medium. A scent conflict can also ulcerate the nasal mucosa (to open up the nasal passage, getting more scent to the olfactory cells), resulting in virtually identical symptoms. A runny nose (from the fluids mentioned above), fever, and swelling, commonly accompany any such repair. A stink conflict can be literal (dog pooped in the kitchen), or figurative (that stinks, I can't take it anymore, I've had it). A scent conflict can involve wanting to catch a whiff of a lost loved one, or smelling trouble, sniffing out a threat. If the symptoms spread, usually down your throat to your lungs, several DHS's, related to the initial stink or scent conflict, are involved, including a sore throat (not wanting to swallow that which figuratively stinks), cough (territorial-fear – see bronchitis above). Other symptoms are typical healing symptoms (headache [EC], and fever).

The tuberculosis bacteria is a cornerstone of the Fourth Biological Law of GNM. It is involved in the removal of temporary cells, provided antibiotics have not disrupted this healing stage. Tuberculosis bacteria can present wherever old-brain (brainstem and cerebellum) directed cell augmentation occurs in the conflict-active (CA) phase, requiring cell removal in the healing phase. Lung, liver, skin, and kidney are common TB sites. The bacteria consume and secrete significant amounts of protein while removing these extra cells. If present in the lungs, this protein is coughed up and spat out as the lungs are cleared of waste cells. It must be replaced through diet. The consequences of not doing so illuminate why the disease was labeled *consumption* in the past. Any long healing phase involving TB bacteria can result in a wasting effect due to protein malnourishment, which can prove fatal.

Asthma manifests as both laryngeal (inhalation) and bronchial (exhalation). The actual asthma attack occurs during the epileptoid crisis (EC) of the SBS. Bronchial asthma involves two DHSs, a territorial-fear conflict in the right hemisphere, which affects the bronchial musculature relay, and a second active conflict in the left hemisphere. The brain relays for the laryngeal muscles mirror the bronchial relays and are in the left hemisphere. A scare-fright conflict is involved here, with a corresponding second DHS on the right hemisphere. When both bronchial and laryngeal muscles are in EC simultaneously, the condition is known as status asthmaticus, which is potentially fatal, depending on the intensity of the DHSs.

Goblet cells in the lungs are responsible for secreting mucus, which moistens and cleans the incoming air. A DHS caused by a fear of not getting enough air (suffocating, drowning, severe asthma attack, etc.)

Healthcare

can cause an initial increase in goblet cells, resulting in more mucus. Cystic fibrosis results from a hanging conflict of this sort. Most, but not all, cases of CF are diagnosed in infants. Could the process of being born, of a possible umbilical cord incident, or too long of a delay in breathing after the mother is no longer supplying her baby oxygen, result in this DHS? The fetus need only subjectively perceive the possibility of suffocation, to the level of a conflict shock. The nature of being a newborn provides the isolative requirement (not being able to share the shock through communication with others) for a DHS, and all that's left is for the SBS to rush to the baby's aid.

In GNM, tumors of the alveoli are linked with a death-fright conflict, and only a death-fright conflict. If smoking causes tumors of the alveoli, then smoking must be part of a DHS wherein the patient has a sudden mortal fear of inhaling tobacco smoke, a fear they internalize; share with no one. In this example, the smoke is the catalyst for the death-fright, not the direct cause. Let me provide another example of a death-fright; receiving a fatal disease diagnosis. I use this to illustrate the intensity required for your brainstem to activate the alveoli growth SBS that a radiologist will later, in the healing phase of the SBS, identify as a pulmonary tumor. There is little chance you (and therefore your doctor) will notice this cell growth in the CA phase, as it is asymptomatic. Not every such diagnosis will result in this DHS, but such is the intensity of the shock necessary to trigger such a reaction.

Secondhand smoke is also implicated in lung cancers. Medical authorities report that 7,300+ people die in this manner yearly.[211] Given that the concentrations of toxins in secondhand smoke are orders of magnitude lower[212] than directly inhaled smoke, either the victims were extraordinarily sensitive to the toxins, or perhaps their fear of the *carcinogenic nature* of the smoke, secondhand or otherwise, resulted in a DHS. I am not advocating the lifting of public smoking bans here; I am merely suggesting that we understand cause before we spend $300+ million per year (see *Appendix*) aiming in what appears to me to be the wrong direction.

Audit

The treatment of lung diseases is a very expensive proposition. Yearly expenditures exceed $3 billion in the USA alone. Mainstream medicine has been researching lung diseases for over a century, with no unequivocal explanations for cause that I could find. Researching for this book has shown me that this is not unusual, as identifying cause does not seem to be the top priority in mainstream medical research, regardless of disease.

If we, as a society, continue down this path, extrapolation predicts refinements in symptom treatment, but also that lung diseases will continue to plague us. This path has been thoroughly explored by now, so I am skeptical that more research along these lines will yield new discoveries as to cause. We can either accept that as our fate or choose to explore new paths.

Mental Illness

Mental illness is a condition that affects a person's thinking, feeling, behavior or mood.

Organization

A prominent medical charity focusing on mental illness was founded in 1979.[213] This grassroots organization has been dedicated to helping Americans affected by mental illness build better lives for almost 40 years.[214] They educate via free programs designed to inform both patient and families. They advocate to shape national policy. They listen via their toll-free telephone service to hundreds of thousands of callers every year looking for guidance, and lastly, they lead public awareness events and activities. Their public policy statement affirms their commitment to finding cures for mental illnesses.[215] They are the foundation for hundreds of state organizations, affiliates, and volunteer leaders. Their revenue for 2016 was $14 million,[216] the bulk of which is covered by private donations.

Funding for mental illness research at the US federal government level is orders of magnitude higher, averaging roughly $3.8 billion per year since 2013 (see *Appendix*). Research thus funded is largely allopathic in nature.[217] Roughly one in six US adults is affected directly by any form of mental illness, with one in 25 being so affected by a serious mental illness.

Mainstream Theory

In their search for a solution to mental illness, what has been the focus of allopathic psychiatry? Mood-altering pharmaceuticals are a pillar of this approach to mental health. Psychotherapy[218] is another tool in the mainstream arsenal, whereby the medical professional uses communication to help a person come to peace with life situations that appear to manifest as mental problems. These first two tools often are used in conjunction by psychiatrists. Intentionally triggering seizures with electroconvulsive therapy is still popular, though nobody seems to understand quite why it works,[219] and we can all breath a little easier given that the fascination with the lobotomy has gone the way of leeches.

Targeting the brain and central nervous system (CNS), pharmaceutical medications address the symptoms of mental illness. As these target organs are arguably the most complex in our bodies, it should come as no surprise that the causes of mental illness remain shrouded. The following is a list of links to conventional medical mental illnesses resources. For the same reasons as in the *Cancer* chapter, I have chosen not to summarize their conclusions. Suffice it to say that the cause of each affliction remains either unknown or unclear.

- Schizophrenia[220]
- Autism[221]
- Bipolar disorder[222]
- Eating disorders[223]
- Borderline personality disorder[224]
- Obsessive-compulsive disorders[225]
- ADHD[226]
- Anxiety[227]
- Psychosis[228]

Healthcare

At this point, I could break down any of the slightly hopeful conclusions in the links above, but as I have already performed a similar exercise, I will simply refer the reader back to the *Cancer* chapter.

There are six main groups of psychiatric medicines[229] to treat and manage mental illness. They all alter the chemistry of an incredibly complex, delicately balanced control system. They were apparently all designed with uncertain knowledge of the cause of the illness they target, and can thus be at best, a valiant attempt to mute the symptoms of what can undoubtedly be devastating conditions. Because of this, it is highly doubtful that any represent a cure, as the chance of finding such in this intricate arena without certain knowledge of cause, is roughly the same as a bull managing to maintain order in a china shop.

- **Antidepressants** treat disorders such as clinical depression, dysthymia, anxiety disorders, eating disorders and borderline personality disorder.
- **Antipsychotics** treat psychotic disorders such as schizophrenia and psychotic symptoms in other conditions such as mood disorders.
- **Anxiolytics** treat anxiety disorders.
- **Depressants** are used as hypnotics, sedatives, and anesthetics.
- **Mood stabilizers** treat bipolar disorder and schizoaffective disorder.
- **Stimulants** treat disorders such as attention deficit hyperactivity disorder (ADHD) and narcolepsy.

Addiction to alcohol is known today as alcohol use disorder, the cause of which is still unknown.[230] Despite this ignorance, there are many efforts to combat this affliction, the most well known of which offers a spiritual path to sobriety, which unfortunately appears to have a success rate of less than 10%.[231] Allopathy provides counseling, rehabilitation (which teaches coping skills), and of course medication to address the symptoms of alcohol dependency. These drugs include:

- **Disulfiram**, which rewards anyone taking it with nausea, vomiting, and headaches anytime they imbibe alcohol. Does nothing to directly address the craving for alcohol.[232]
- **Naltrexone**, which is used after alcohol detoxification. This drug interferes with brain chemistry by blocking receptors thought to be associated with the alcohol *high*.[233]
- **Acamprosate**, the latest drug approved for alcohol use disorder, the US Department of Health and Human Services is unsure how the drug actually works, postulating that it may reduce withdrawal symptoms.[234]

Maverick Theory

Mental illness, according to GNM, occurs when two or more active phase (CA or EC) SBSs are running simultaneously in opposing halves of the brain. Dr. Hamer referred to this as a constellation. The SBS (reaction to DHS) directs your body to a particular action, in a specific direction. When there is more than one active SBS, the separate directions may conflict, may interfere with each other, causing the symptoms of mental illness. Understand that all SBSs are intended to bring about a positive biological advantage. The combinations and sequence of the SBSs in forming a constellation determines the symptoms. It is the collision of these programs that cause the observed symptoms we call mental illness.

This straightforward definition points to an immediate solution: relief from the symptoms of mental illness requires resolving conflicts

Healthcare

so that no more than one SBS remains active. Given it is safe to do so, certainly zero SBSs are preferable to even one, however, as it pertains to mental illness, reduction to one SBS will suffice. The order in which the conflicts are resolved can be a critical consideration, best determined by an experienced GNM health consultant. Should a conflict that triggered an SBS that comprises part of a constellation be resolved, then that SBS will enter the second, or healing, phase and can naturally introduce its own physical symptoms.

Constellations are inferred by observing symptoms and confirmed by CT scans, where multiple active HHs can be detected. Here we have the cause of the illness, the reasons for the symptoms, and the path back to health.

Mental Illness
- **DHS** (conflict shock) Multiple unresolved active conflicts.
- **SBS** (2-phase reaction to DHS) Unique case.
    - There is no specific SBS that relates to mental illness
    - Most of the many types of mental illness result from the brain attempting to respond to two (or more) conflict shocks with opposite or conflicting responses.
- **HH** (concentric ring pattern) On both brain hemispheres.
- **CA** (SBS phase 1) All mental illness symptoms occur in CA phase
    - Hypersensitivity (paranoia, acrophobia, auditory hallucinations) sensory part of both sides of the brain involved at once.
    - Psychosis (panic/anxiety, anorexia, catatonia) being directed by the two hemispheres of the cerebral cortex to deal with life situations that call for opposite reactions.

- Sociopathy (feeling of complete absence of emotion) results specifically from a pair of conflicts handled by certain positions on either side of the cerebellum.
- **PCL** Not applicable.

To give an idea of how GNM sees mental illness, consider the following examples. These are not meant as diagnosis, as any such should be rendered by a qualified professional. They are intended merely to highlight links between common conflicts and defined mental conditions.

Alcoholism[235] is seen as a combination of an existence conflict (kidney collecting tubules) and a fluid conflict (*literal*: near drowning, *figurative*: cash flow, liquidity), affecting the kidney parenchyma.

GNM views anxiety as a combination of a danger conflict, such as heading into a potentially dangerous situation, and a powerlessness conflict wherein you perceive yourself as helpless or not in control. The first results in an HH in the branchial arch relay and the second in an HH in the thyroid duct relay.

Depression and mania result from territorial conflict constellations. There are five territorial relays in each cerebral hemisphere which respond to four conflicts to produce depression. These conflicts are territorial (fear, loss, anger, and boundary). Mania or depression is determined by what Dr. Hamer called the Scale Rules. If the left hemisphere is suffering the greater weight conflict, mania will ensue, if the right hemisphere is thus targeted, depression will be the outcome.

Eating disorders such as anorexia are viewed as any active conflict in the left territory conflict area of the brain coupled with an HH in the (right hemisphere) stomach, bile duct, bulbous duodeni, or pancreas duct relay.

Self-injury (cutting) involves a cerebellum constellation (worry conflict in both hemispheres) which manifests as an emotional void. Couple this with constellations resulting in thoughts of death (post mortal constellation), or anger (bio-aggressive constellation) and you have the ingredients for a textbook case of self-harm.

Constellations of the visual cortex (active conflicts in both halves) result in paranoia, or persecution mania. The visual cortex is responsible for seeing the potential threat, as the paranoid *sees* a threat behind every tree. A persecution conflict coupled with the conflicts responsible for anxiety can lead to a feeling of being cornered.

Audit

The understanding of the mind is unquestionably in its early stages. This should be expected. As Lyall Watson concluded: "If the brain were so simple we could understand it, we would be so simple we couldn't." This complexity, and the understandable relative ignorance thereof, really should dictate that of all the systems of the body that can malfunction, this is the candidate most in need of a wide arc of different medical approaches. To me, this is the field where putting all of your eggs into one basket makes the least sense.

It is also a field of medicine that offers a wide range of very down to earth, easy to understand, hints into the nature of some of its illnesses, and absolutely none as to why others occur. It is easy to understand that depression could easily settle into a person who has suffered a devastating personal loss. It is far more difficult to understand why someone might hear voices in their head goading them to commit crimes.

I think it safe to say that most of us have been depressed. Far fewer, however, have been clinically depressed, although it makes sense that the causes could be the same, if not in degree, then certainly in kind. Just how this manifests as clinical depression is still unclear to all but GNM, which not only provides a definition why depressions occur, but has fully defined depressive versus manic conditions, and can even correctly diagnose them by studying a patients brain CT scan.

The mainstream solution to mental illness is a maintenance plan. Symptoms are managed, often for a lifetime, while the patient struggles with side effects, some of them allegedly dangerous to society.[236] The cost of such a plan can be enormous, while the best that too many of its patients can expect is a mere numbing or dulling of symptoms.[237]

Alternative solutions face the same obstacles that the mainstream approach does, as the mind is incredibly complex, and no medicine, except perhaps time, will overcome life events. It too struggles to identify the cause of these conditions, although by casting a truly wide net, it has explored previously uncharted areas of mental healthcare.[238]

GNM offers the only precise definition of mental illness I have ever read. By mapping brain constellations, it can correctly diagnose conditions from CT brain scans alone. It is the only medical paradigm I am aware of that draws an unmistakable connection between mental and physical illness, identifying mental illness as a logical result of collisions in the progression of subconscious programs aiding an individual in overcoming acute psychological shock. This original insight leads to the startling conclusion that apart from addressing the individual conflict shocks, no other treatment is necessary for

Healthcare

overcoming mental illness; that the symptoms are the byproduct of multiple active shocks and will naturally disappear once the underlying individual conflicts are resolved. This would imply that in GNM, mental illness is essentially treated as a *buy one get one free* sort of arrangement, where once the underlying problem is addressed, the secondary effect, the mental illness, will disappear on its own.

In practice, things tend not to be so cut and dry, and mental illness symptoms may require more immediate, albeit by their nature temporary, direct attention. An inescapable difficulty in treating a patient suffering from mental illness with GNM lies in its participatory requirement. Informed dialog is the GNM practitioners main tool. Depending on the illness and its severity, this patient requirement may not be achievable. As recommended, earlier, it is best to understand and choose your medical options while you are well.

Pancreas

This chapter deals with disorders of the pancreas other than cancer (see *Cancer* chapter).

Diabetes is an umbrella term for diseases where impaired regulation results in high levels of blood sugar.

Pancreatitis is an inflammation of the pancreas.

Organization

The most prominent medical charity focusing on pancreas health was founded 77 years ago in 1940.[239] They are the largest private US health charity funding diabetes research. They seek to prevent and cure diabetes, while working to improve the lives of those touched by the disease. They are organized into roughly 90 local offices throughout the United States. Their revenue for 2016 was $171,062,000,[240] the bulk of which is covered by private donations and funds raised at special events. Roughly 80,000 people in the USA die from the disease yearly, placing it eighth on the leading cause of death list. The annual (2016 data) global economic cost of diabetes alone is estimated to be $825 billion.[241]

Organizations dedicated to the pancreas in general, not specifically diabetes or pancreatic cancers, are relatively small.

Healthcare

Funding for diabetes research at the US federal government level is far higher than at private charities (see *Appendix*). That this is so, becomes clear, given estimates of more than 100 million (roughly one in three) US citizens having either active or pre-diabetes.[242]

Mainstream Theory

The cause of diabetes (all forms) is not well understood[243] by mainstream medicine at present. Researchers are predictably focusing on environmental influences and genes, as specific pathogens have been noticeably absent in the search for a culprit. This mimics the path taken by allopathy for many other diseases, and will presumably lead to similar frustration in pinpointing cause. It's been a while, so I'll repeat my assertion: if you don't understand cause, you're trusting that dumb luck will correct the problem. Let's see how lucky mainstream medicine has been in getting a handle on diabetes.

Allopathy is here, once again, reduced to managing a disease, attempting to control its symptoms, while patients are left to hope that Nature will correct the problems, so they can get back to having more than one wish. Despite a survey[244] of monetary donors for type 1 diabetes showing that 96% wanted their money to spent on cure research, apparently, only about 7% is actually spent in that area.[245] A portion of that 7% is dedicated to creating a reliable artificial pancreas, which is no *cure* at all, but rather an automated symptom management system. It seems the notion that Nature has failed yet again is alive and kicking in this allopathic circle as well. All the while, the global rate of new diabetes cases continues to rise.

Mainstream medicine opines that pancreatitis is the result of improperly activated digestive enzymes.[246] Apparently these enzymes activate while still in the pancreas. Completely missing, as far as I could find, is an explanation why they would do so and just how that would be biologically advantageous.

Maverick Theory

The pancreas produces digestive enzymes as well as hormones that control blood sugar and stomach acid levels. These secretions serve three distinct purposes, are controlled from three separate locations in the brain, and thus react to three distinct conflict shocks. The pancreatic gland produces digestive enzymes, derives from the endoderm and is thus controlled from the brainstem, as are all gastrointestinal tract organs and their evolutionary derivatives. The pancreatic ducts connect the pancreas to the intestine through the duodenum, derive from the ectoderm, and are thus controlled by the cerebral cortex. The islet cells produce hormones that regulate blood sugar (alpha islet cells produce glucagon, which controls the liver production of glucose, and beta islet cells produce insulin which governs liver uptake of glucose), derive from the ectoderm and are thus also controlled by the cerebral cortex.

Since the pancreatic gland itself produces digestive enzymes, morsel conflicts (indigestible morsels) can result in the production of extra pancreatic cells to aid in the digestion of that morsel. In predators, such a conflict might arise after swallowing too large of a bone fragment, which then lodges in the intestine, threatening the animal's life. A flood of enzymes to digest the bone quickly is the correct biological response, amplified by extra enzyme-producing cells. In humans, conflicts of this type are almost always abstract in nature and are often a result of angry family quarrels – arguments that are *hard to digest*. Disagreements over money, inheritance, duty, etc., are linked to this morsel conflict. As with all old-brain controlled cells, augmentation occurs during the active phase of a conflict. Hanging-active conflicts can result in a sufficiently large enough growth to be called a tumor. Tumor growth rate is determined by the intensity of the conflict. Mainstream medicine interprets faster rates as malignant, while slower rates are interpreted as benign. Upon conflict resolution, fungi and mycobacteria remove the extra cells, which is usually accompanied by pain and swelling. If there are not sufficient cells to be classified a tumor, mainstream medicine calls this healing phase pancreatitis.

Conflicts that affect the cerebral cortex first result in an ulceration of cells, followed upon conflict resolution by a reversal, or production of new cells. Pancreatic ducts respond to a territorial-anger conflict (in males), or an identity conflict (in females), by ulcerating, becoming wider, to accommodate an increase in the flow of pancreatic fluids into the duodenum. This improves metabolism which then results in more immediate energy to resolve the conflict.

A territorial-anger conflict is one of several territory conflicts GNM has identified, with the others being territorial-fear, territorial-loss, and territorial-marking. The following example illustrates a general territory conflict. Many animals in nature are not loners but naturally gravitate towards social groupings (herds, packs, etc.). This instinct has several advantages: safety in numbers from outside aggression, distribution of the responsibility and success in finding food, and warning of attack. These social constructs often share a typical structure. Among males, there is one who is dominant, from a combination of physical strength, cunning, endurance, determination, attitude. We designate this individual the alpha male. Think of him as a king, or a boss, or a president of their particular group. The area he roams is his territory, as are its resources (at least the ones that interest him). The rest of the group is his responsibility (especially the breeding females), and can also be seen as his territory. Any threat to this territory can trigger a territorial conflict in the alpha male. A territorial-anger conflict would be, as the name suggests, one wherein a threat to the territory invokes anger, one to be met with force. This often arises from theft or attempted theft. So in my alpha male example, a challenge to his authority, an attempt to steal his crown so to speak, might result in this type of DHS. In humans, these territories are often the home, the job, the school, the family, the town, the country.

An identity conflict refers to being unable to establish one's place, one's position. In animal groups, a pecking order is established, and a conflict that threatens that order would be of this type. In human societies, there are female queens, bosses and presidents, positions of authority that in the animal world mostly fall to males. This human reality, however, is a conscious phenomenon, and GNM deals with subconscious reactions, based presumably on countless eons of evolution, much of which is common to all animals. With rare exceptions, the group head is the dominant group member, and that role mostly falls to a male. This is not a value judgment, simply an observation. So when a GNM practitioner evaluates a patient with symptoms indicating an issue with the pancreatic ducts, they would first look to either territorial-anger conflicts if the patient were male, or identity conflicts if the patient were female.

Pancreatic islet cells are responsible for hormones that control blood sugar. Alpha cells produce glucagon, and beta cells produce insulin. Glucagon prompts the liver to create glucose from stored glycogen, increasing blood sugar levels. Insulin prompts the liver to create glycogen from glucose, reducing blood sugar levels. They are functional opposites. Glucose is absorbed directly into the blood by the small intestine from the digestion of starches and complex sugars. One of the functions of the liver is to act as a repository of this sugar (as glycogen). If you overeat glucose producing food, insulin is created which directs the liver to store the excess. If you undereat glucose producing food, glucagon is created which directs the liver to convert stored glycogen into glucose.

The DHS linked to the alpha cells is fear-revulsion, a shock involving loathing. A drop in glucagon will decrease blood sugar by constricting the release of reserves. Declining blood sugar levels trigger, among other symptoms, a craving for sweets, (to provide an instant boost of muscle fuel), and the jitters, to better flee the situation, if necessary.

The DHS linked to the beta cells is fear-resistance, a shock involving a feeling of *I don't want to do this*. A drop in insulin will increase blood sugar by not triggering the storage of reserves. Increasing blood sugar levels makes the sugar instantly available for use by muscles, to better resist. An unresolved conflict of this type will result in consistently elevated blood sugar levels, with all of its accompanying symptoms, and a diagnosis of diabetes.

Complications arising in the epileptic crisis (EC) with islet cell conflicts can be fatal, as rapid and extreme changes in blood sugar level can lead to diabetic coma, which must be treated quickly.

Audit

The United States spends more than $1 billion per year in response to pancreatic issues. Globally, 422 million people suffered from diabetes alone in 2014, up from 108 million in 1980.[247] There has not been a fourfold increase in the population in those years, so a combination of better diagnostics and an actual escalation in the disease rate seems to be responsible. Obviously, the mainstream approach has not been successful in lowering the incidences of this debilitating disease. This sad fact should by now come as no surprise given the poor understanding of cause. The medical consequences of abnormal blood sugar levels alone are catastrophic enough, being directly implicated in blindness, kidney failure, heart attacks, stroke and lower limb amputation. Disease management is a pale substitute for a functioning pancreas but unfortunately seems to be all that mainstream medicine can offer at present.

Alternative medicine also chases symptoms concerning illnesses of the pancreas, and while there have been successes, they too, have no clear understanding of cause. Sorry to sound like a broken record here, but I've got to go where the facts lead.

GNM again, unambiguously explains cause, thereby suggesting what is required so that Nature can restore the health of your pancreas. Clearly, if this can be achieved, artificial symptom management becomes unnecessary. Not only does GNM present an understanding of blood sugar disorders, but also of duct and gland disorders, all the while offering concise physical evidence in the form of tracking HH development on CT scans for all stages of illness. Why GNM is at best ignored in the face of this runaway epidemic is, to me, unfathomable.

Skin

This chapter deals with disorders of the skin other than cancer (see *Cancer* chapter).

There are scores of identified skin diseases. They either affect the outer layer that we see called the epidermis, or a thicker inner layer underlying the epidermis called the dermis, or corium skin.

Organization

The largest professional association for doctors specializing in diseases of the skin was founded nearly 80 years ago in 1938[248]. It represents roughly 18,000 dermatologists, with total revenues for 2015 reaching $44,149,554.[249]

I have been unable to find another large-scale organization for skin issues per se. This seems to be because other organizations pursuit of a cure often includes skin. Skin cancers are wrapped up into cancer institutes. Sexually transmitted diseases are wrapped into infectious disease institutes. Likewise, childhood illnesses like measles are covered by vaccines. This leaves mostly nonfatal diseases, and as such the organizations that spring up to deal with them are relatively small.

Federal expenditures on just skin issues are also relatively small, and I have found no simple way of breaking out just skin research from other categories (see *Appendix*). And yet, a surprisingly large number of

Skin

diseases of the skin have been identified by mainstream medicine, as it is our most visible organ. It is for this reason I have included this separate chapter.

Mainstream Theory

The causes of skin disease remain mostly unclear to allopathy, though fungus, virus, bacteria, genes, autoimmune reactions, and insect bites head the list of suspects. Below is an incomplete list of such diseases.[250]

Athletes foot, acne, basalioma, boils, candidiasis of the skin, cellulitis, chancroid, chickenpox, cowpox, dermatitis, eczema, gonorrhea, herpes, hives, ichthyosis, impetigo, Kaposi sarcoma, keloids, leprosy, lichen planus, lupus erythematosus, melasma, measles, melanoma, monkeypox, mouth ulcers, nail fungus, Netherton syndrome, pemphigoid, psoriasis, rash, ringworm, rosacea, rubella, scabies, scarlet fever, scleroderma, shingles, skin cysts, smallpox, syphilis, tinea versicolor, vitiligo, warts.

Allopathic treatments for skin diseases attributed to fungus are often only initially successful. The fungus may return time and again seemingly regardless of how careful you are to avoid it. If an external fungus that attacks your skin is responsible for athlete's foot, why does it stop at mainly the sole of the foot; why not the top of the foot too? Why are not athlete's ankle or athlete's leg or athlete's body just as common as athlete's foot? Perhaps there is another explanation for these types of skin problems?

Allopaths treat some skin problems attributed to viruses with vaccines, especially diseases of childhood. Yet it seems[251] that there is

169

quite a bit of admittedly anecdotal evidence that vaccination is not the panacea public service announcements would have us believe. Smallpox was thought eradicated by vaccine, and still, people complain of symptoms that in another era would have resulted in a diagnosis of smallpox. Today, these cases are diagnosed as pustular eczema, or if you live in Africa, monkeypox.[252] A wide range of questionable diagnoses accompanies many skin diseases. Measles is one such example: rubella, erythema infectiosum, exanthem subitum, primary HIV, infectious mononucleosis, medications, scarlet fever, and pneumonia are possible alternative diagnoses.[253] What biases are in play, even if just subconsciously, if a doctor knows that their patient is showing symptoms of a disease against which they have previously been vaccinated?

A favorite allopathic explanation for diseases for which no pathogen is present is that the body is somehow confused and has either misprogrammed genes or is attacking itself. Members of this *autoimmune* or *confused body* category include the skin diseases psoriasis, scleroderma, and systemic lupus erythematosus. Why the body should attack itself is again unclear.[254] How that would be biologically advantageous is not explained. Consider the following maverick theories of skin health issues, and understand that the mainstream interpretation of the facts requires you to accept that Nature has failed spectacularly in what is estimated to be roughly 5-7% of the US population (figures for all autoimmune diseases, not just skin).[255] This number has increased steadily over time,[256] indicating either better diagnostics or that Nature is becoming increasingly incompetent in fulfilling her primary goal with respect to humans.

Finding genetic anomalies in people diagnosed with a specific disease is like finding bacteria at disease sites. Did the bacteria cause the disease, or is there another reason for their presence? Did the genetic differences cause the problem, or does that which controls genes (the brain), have ulterior motives? Is the body attacking itself for no reason, or is it that we don't understand the reason for the symptoms we see?

Maverick Theory

Dr. Hamer was of the opinion that all diseases of the epidermis result from separation conflicts and that all diseases of the dermis result from attack conflicts. Sometimes fungus is involved and sometimes bacteria, but only ever in the second or healing phase, thus eliminating them as possible causal agents (logically cannot be causal if absent until PCL). Genetic markers are also occasionally present, but as they are not static entities, as they are under the control of the brain, one cannot rewind time to before the illness to inspect them, and therefore I conclude that they too are not causal (until proven otherwise). I have already written enough about the elusive virus, so no more on that topic.

A separation conflict is one that involves a loss of touch, of contact, with the skin. This loss can be either unwanted or desired. An example of an unwanted loss conflict is a child having to attend daycare or school for the first time, being forced to separate from their parents. Embryology has shown conclusively that the sensory cortex (part of the new-brain) controls the epidermis, indicating initial cell loss, followed after conflict resolution by cell gain. This cell loss manifests as a loss of touch-sense, or numbness, a meaningful biological response to lessen the blow of having to touch and feel new things rather than the comfort of the familiar. If and when the child acclimates to their new surroundings, the conflict is resolved, and healing can begin. This involves cell growth and a return of touch-sense. In the chapter *Kidneys and Bladder*, I explained the GNM discovery of KCTS. Since this scenario could very easily be perceived as an abandonment situation, this child may very well have both SBS's active (abandonment in CA [first phase of SBS], separation in PCL [second phase of SBS]), which would amplify, and thus complicate, the healing symptoms. Measles, chickenpox, rubella and scarlet fever are all *diseases* this child might develop.

An unwanted separation conflict might arise from not wanting to be kissed, or apprehension that you might *catch something* from a sexual partner. During the conflict-active phase, the same initial cell loss would occur as in the above example, followed, upon conflict resolution, with cell growth. As all cell growth occurs in a liquid medium, and such a state on the epidermis would not be physically possible, blisters form to trap the liquid from the effects of gravity, thus enabling healing. Once the EC completes, and the fluid is expelled, the blisters collapse into scabs. This example person would most likely be diagnosed with Herpes in the case of the kiss, or a venereal disease in the other example.

A separation conflict can also lead to hair loss if the ulceration is deep enough. This problem is so widespread that well over $1 billion is spent annually[257] addressing it in the United Staes alone.

Psoriasis, the cause of which is still unclear to allopathy,[258] is explained by GNM as two separation conflicts manifesting in the same location: one in the active stage, and one in the healing stage.

The cerebellum (a part of the old-brain) controls the corium skin. Thus, the conflict-active (CA) period will be marked by cell growth, followed by ulceration upon conflict resolution, the opposite of conflicts affecting the epidermis. A DHS affecting the corium skin is referred to by GNM as an attack conflict. These attacks can be felt concretely, as in actual physical attack or felt abstractly, such as hurtful words. Being exposed to things considered filthy can also be perceived as an attack.

Skin

While the conflict is active, the corium skin thickens at the perceived impact point, increasing its protective properties. When the conflict is resolved, the excess cells are removed by microbes, resulting in, among other things, a foul smell. If tuberculosis bacteria are involved, a conventional doctor would render a diagnosis of skin tuberculosis.

As an example, prolonged exposure to the sun in light-skinned people results in melanin production, a dark pigment that protects the dermis from UV rays. Dark-skinned people produce melanin regardless of the sun's exposure. Mainstream medicine sees melanoma as DNA damage caused by excessive exposure to the sun. Allopathy theorizes that this damaged DNA causes the skin cells to run amok, destroying healthy cells in their path.

A GNM explanation of this scenario involves a subconscious desire for more protection than melanin can provide, and so the corium skin, which borders the melanin-producing melanocyte cells, thickens. In effect, the first line of defense was deemed inadequate, and so the second line, just beneath it, is activated. Once the conflict is resolved, the new dermis cells are ulcerated, which is admittedly not pleasant. However, attempting to remove the ulcerations with surgery may lead to further attack conflicts near the site (depending on how the surgery is perceived), creating a vicious cycle that sees the melanoma *spread*. Ignorance of the cause of the melanoma, coupled with the common perception of attacking germs or rogue cells, might also contribute to a sense of assault, with similar results. An understanding of GNM may alter the perception of these *attacks* and hopefully avert a DHS.

Smallpox is theorized by allopathy to be caused by the variola major virus, with the telltale lesions developing from capillaries in the dermis[259]. Native North American populations were decimated by this disease as European settlers pushed west. GNM explains the sores as

173

the healing phase of an attack conflict, followed by large numbers of deaths from pneumonia, which is attributed to a territorial-fear conflict and exacerbated by an existence conflict, which can cause the kidneys to retain water, thus amplifying healing symptoms.

A common corium skin issue elegantly explained by GNM is foot fungus or athlete's foot. The sweat glands reside in the corium skin. If contact with something that is perceived to be filthy, something from which the body requires protection (for instance a public shower floor), raises to the level of a DHS, the resulting cell augmentation will include more sweat glands on the sole, not the top of the foot, nor the ankle, nor the leg. Sweat is useful for cooling the skin, but also for cleaning it by washing away unwanted contact. These added sweat producing cells increase the effectiveness of cleaning the soiled area. When the conflict is resolved, fungi or bacteria remove the extra cells, resulting in an unpleasant smell. If the patient is ignorant of this process, they may perceive this as more filth, another attack, and so the cycle continues.

Acne is another common corium skin issue. An estimated 500 million people are affected globally. While this is usually considered a mild disease, I want to illustrate the GNM explanation and contrast it to my understanding of the allopathic explanation. Acne affects mainly the face and back, two targets linked with the phrases *losing face* and *get off my back*. Acne also primarily affects teenagers, people navigating the sometimes rocky path to adulthood, where they are often unsure of their social standing and where criticism can easily be perceived as an attack. Cell growth occurs during the active phase (CA) to better protect the area under attack. The healing phase of such conflicts ushers in a reversal of this growth, culminating in inflammation and pus (the pimple), which, if subjected to ridicule, may create more of the same conflicts. Allopathy links acne with puberty, though it acknowledge that acne is not exclusive to adolescence. It explains the telltale pimples as hair follicles clogged with dead skin cells and oil, but resorts to risk factors to explain why this should not be a lifelong affliction, as dead skin cells and oil are not exclusive to puberty. Perhaps cognizant of these issues, allopathy's fall back position is faulty genes.[260] While genes may be responsible, Occam's razor suggests otherwise.

Audit

There are more cataloged diseases of the skin than any other organ. A report was released in 2013 claiming that skin diseases wreak an expensive yearly toll in the form of lost productivity ($11 billion) and treatment ($75 billion), touching roughly one in four Americans.[261]

This is no minor area of disease, as the over-the-counter market of lotions and salves in any supermarket can attest. I suppose that the exposed nature of skin has much to do with that, enabling a thriving slather-based DIY therapy regimen. Adding to that, the worldwide daily tally of sexually transmitted infections (STIs) exceeds 1 million, and while some are not diseases of the skin, many are.[262] Forced mandatory vaccines policies have spawned resistance movements that unite government overreach watchdogs and medical freedom activists around the globe. And yet all of these treatments, seem to at best, address symptoms.

That is, except GNM. Basing its conclusions on embryology, it has identified two, and only two causes responsible for the myriad of skin diseases cataloged by mainstream medicine. For the epidermis, a separation conflict lies at the root, and for the dermis, an attack conflict. Why is this concept, so easy to test, ignored, and even outlawed (illegal practice of medicine, wherein unproven methods are used) by the medical establishment? I have my suspicions; I expect you do too.

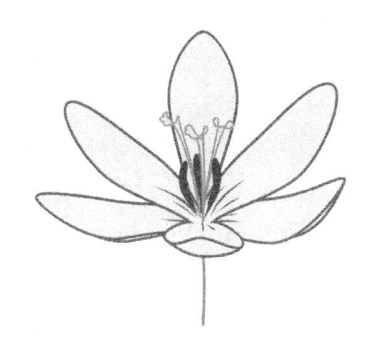

Conclusion

Patient Hat

My conclusions in this matter are in part driven by the actual record the mainstream approach to health has compiled over the past 100 years or so. The allopathic paradigm has been around for longer, but only rose to its dominant position in the past century.[263] If I have appeared upset, or incredulous at times, I can only offer that it was the data that drove those emotions. To be frank, I don't understand how anyone could look at the data and not react in that way. Illness is something that will affect every single person at least once in their lives, often drastically; we should all strive for the truth.

All of us are given a metaphorical *patient hat* at birth. We *wear* it when sick. For the unfortunate among us, it is well worn. A relative few are given a second hat to wear later in life, that of healthcare industry employee. The first hat is mandatory, the second, voluntary, an important distinction. A healthcare industry employee may champion their company's efforts in the healthcare space, be rightfully proud of the work they do, and yet, may face a dilemma when forced to wear their first hat, when they take ill. For then, there is no room for the trappings of business, no conflict between health and career, there is only the truth, and Nature will have her way, every time. Let us suppose that this person's career just happens to align with their illness; say they work for a dialysis machine manufacturer and are diagnosed with early stage renal failure. This machine, though it has prolonged many lives, is a pale substitute for a functioning kidney. In that moment of truth, for that patient, the rubber truly meets the road.

As I mentioned in the introduction, Nature is indifferent; she will not listen to your pleas, should your preferred medical strategy prove not up to the task of returning your health. She will not bend to accommodate your career, your assumptions, your worldview. It is for you to bend to her if you would see your health return. That hard reality ought to direct all medical progress, but sadly that does not always appear to be the case. For example, how many allopathic oncologists would refuse chemotherapy and radiation (for certain cancers) for themselves or their family, the very procedures they recommend for strangers? The question is nuanced, but as it turns out, quite a few.[264] Why? Does it have something to do with a realization I alluded to earlier: that they alone (or their loved ones) must make this mandatory journey, not their industry, not their hospital, not their peers or their boss? At that point, career loyalty will take a back seat to the truth. Everybody wearing that first hat has no time for the many wishes, including career. All are focused on the one wish, as Nature demands.

In this book, I have explored many medical charities whose stated purpose is to eradicate their target illness. All of them favor the mainstream medical approach. Not one of them has found success, by which I mean: organize to eliminate a disease, raise capital to fund research towards this goal, master the disease, its cause, and cure, and finally shutter their doors, as their purpose has been fulfilled – not one. The first two steps are where it stops. By their own admission, the clear discovery of cause in the third step remains elusive, while cure, which would trigger the fourth and final step has yet to be achieved. You would think, after all this time, if their's were a viable path, that at least one of these organizations would have reached the finish line by now.

What progress has been made, seems to be focused on the treatment of symptoms. Is the search for cause even a top priority? A couple of these organizations have been exploring this apparently cause-meager

Conclusion

path for more than a century, and most have been around for scores of years. Charitable contributions to medical causes in the past century far exceed $1 trillion in the USA alone.[265] Federal government medical research departments have spent many times that amount; worldwide, the amount is still higher. Much of this money was presumably spent on research into mainstream solutions. They have been dogged in their search, pressing on where others would have stopped, like a government department backed by a never-ending stream of taxation. I can only wonder if it has occurred to them that perhaps they are on the wrong road. If their's is the correct path, surely I can be forgiven for expecting that by now, with that much backing, that the cause of a (former) major killer disease would be unambiguously clear.

And yet, if the public wishes to fund such pursuits, it is their money, freely given, and I can find no fault in that. Unless of course, it is to highlight the fact that doctors who choose to operate outside of mainstream medical boundaries too often find themselves the targets of litigation. Some of these doctors are pursuing the same stated goals of the mainstream but are using other roads. These alternatives to the status quo (Hamer, Rife, Naessens, Clark, Hoxley, Burzynski, to name but a few)[266] are hounded in legal courtrooms, at great expense (which the profitable mainstream can comfortably afford, whereas the upstart typically cannot), in the name of public safety. Who is initiating this litigation, who was the architect of the laws these upstarts are supposedly violating, and who ultimately is funding all of this?[267] From my spectator's perspective, this looks like a lopsided turf war. Where does regard for the truth figure in all of this?

If medicine is a science then, by definition, all those who embrace it must accept that better theories exist and are waiting to be discovered. Who is to say that a better theory cannot be radically different from, and outside of, the status quo? Why must it be somebody in the mainstream who discovers it? Mainstream medicine itself changes course from within from time to time (recall any major advance: antibiotics, X-rays, etc.). Some of these discoveries were radical enough as to require the adoption of new axioms (gene theory is but one example). To me, the problem seems to be one of control, in a word, bureaucracy. Well, perhaps that is a necessary part of so large an organization, but I've got to say, from where I stand, it sure looks like it's getting in the way, while millions of people are still suffering and dying. Perhaps such staunch control should wait until medicine has made substantial progress understanding cause in category F (heart disease, cancer, diabetes, etc.), and stands on firmer theoretical ground.

Is every alternative medical paradigm effective and safe? Certainly not, but neither is the mainstream, a perhaps inconvenient observation that anyone paying even the slightest attention can easily see (e.g. prescription drug possible side effect warnings).[268] It hardly seems reasonable to me, to implement a virtual legal monopoly in medicine when there is still so much that is clearly not understood. Given mainstream medical experts own assessments, that the cause of disease is still uncertain, why stifle any research? Why block any road? Why rip families apart for the offense of refusing to subject their children to a medical paradigm the parents understandably mistrust?[269] Do we not, as a society, want the truth here? We are all in the same boat. Nobody wants to be sick, not even a little.

That such behavior is tolerated, indeed encouraged, is a sad testament to the public's understanding of a most precious gift, their good health. *Politics has no place in medicine* is a familiar cry, and I agree. Some would go so far as to say profit has no place, though I would contend that since we all have bills to pay, regulating health care to hobby status is a bad idea. Profit, regardless of what else it might be, is a powerful motivator.

Status Quo

Health insurance today (2017) is practically unaffordable.[270] You either receive it as part of your job, along with salary, or you qualify for medical welfare. Everyone not in one of those two pots is screwed. Those on the low end of the salary scale are denied employer health benefits for this reason – it is simply too expensive. Basic catastrophic health insurance (with sky-high deductibles) for a family can cost more than many mortgages. Religious health share organizations are far more affordable but carry with them specific requirements, and so may not be for everyone. As more people cannot afford the premiums, this will only increase cost pressure on the remaining insurance payers, as the Emergency Treatment and Labor Act, which guarantees ER treatment regardless of ability to pay, has always been an unfunded mandate.[271] Let an illness go untreated long enough, and there is a good chance it will result in an ER visit. Mandated health benefits for full-time work (Affordable Care Act) all but assures fewer available full-time positions. Political maneuvering aside, this tremendous cost either destroys full-time jobs or threatens to bankrupt the payer (employer or individual); there is no third choice that I can see. That people will continue to get sick, is a given. That we must somehow deal with a cost that is exploding upward, is a direct result of the mainstream medical system in place today. In this system, the cause of illness is seemingly irrelevant, and expensive, often lifelong maintenance, is the rule. The situation is frightening. It will either radically change, or I fear it will bankrupt everybody it touches.[272] Every other medical paradigm outlined in this book is considerably cheaper than the current mainstream. That they are not embraced, that they are often not covered by existing insurance plans,[273] if for nothing more than cost savings, is to me inexplicable.

Everything in Nature happens for a reason. That does not mean we are automatically privy to it. Finding reasons for medical issues can clearly be difficult, but medical ignorance should be a welcomed clue to look elsewhere for answers. If you have learned there are no answers to be had down a path, why waste any more precious time looking in that direction? A given medical paradigm's axioms are theirs, not yours. You are free to question them, even to reject them, if they ring false to you. If everyone did that, medical competition alone would take a huge bite out of costs, as monopolies naturally have no incentive to lower costs. A *no cure* prognosis to a *fatal* disease is a clear warning that your doctor is tapped out, that there are no more ideas to be had from that source, and is a strong prediction that death awaits you in the near future should you not change course. What should you do if faced with that scenario? Well, I can't imagine a more personal decision. If you continue, your doctor says you will die. If you go home (given that you can), you could suffer more before passing. If you refuse to accept the death sentence, and continue to search for health, where do you look?

This is often when the accusations of predatory medicine are leveled, when alternatives to the status quo are labeled *quack* by the proponents of the mainstream. All I see in those situations are sour grapes. Why should you not continue to look for a reason for your illness? Why automatically assume that since the mainstream has no answers, that none exist? To help answer those questions, consider that the evidence presented in this book casts serious doubt on the mainstream understanding of the cause of many, if not most, diseases. Are their protests then, in these situations, reasonable? Unlike Bastiat's Superman[274], mainstream doctors are not made of a finer clay, wise to answers that escape the rest of us. If they were, they would never get

Conclusion

chronically sick. They are expert in their field, but that does not make them expert in all matters health. There are plenty of dead-ends in medicine, but I am convinced there are clear reasons for all illnesses; I believe they can be found. Actually, I think somebody already has.

How does a doctor successfully intervene and *cure* a patient in most medical paradigms? I'm talking about category F illnesses only here (cancer, diabetes, MS, etc.). Well, each modality will have their own approach, as will each disease, so I can only generalize, but in my experience as a patient, it proceeds something like this:

You notice something wrong and visit your doctor. They examine you, subjecting you to whatever tests their particular field employs. If allopathic, the tests tend to be technical (CT scan, MRI, etc.) and atomistic. If alternative, the tests are more varied, but also generally holistic. If maverick, the testing will often be an optional brain CT scan and focused dialog, trying to identify a past conflict shock that is associated with your symptoms. A diagnosis will determine your doctor's course of action. If allopathic, drugs (patent or otherwise) or surgery will often be employed. These will mostly target the symptoms of the illness. If alternative, a similar course of action will ensue, with different (usually herbal) drugs. One can expect less focus on surgery and more on diet and lifestyle recommendations. If maverick, there will be a focus on cause (DHS), the biological meaning of the SBS, timeline or which phase of the SBS you are in, conflict resolution, track avoidance, and potential EC complications. A KCTS will be ruled out or dealt with immediately. Drugs and surgery may play a role, but always subservient to a conscious understanding of what is happening (cause). In all cases, Nature will correct the problem or not. The efforts of any medical paradigm will either interfere with or make this process more comfortable, as Nature alone can restore health, catastrophic emergency procedures notwithstanding.

GNM

For me, the solution that best answers the questions I posed in the introduction is German New Medicine. Since I am on the outside looking in (to repeat: I am not a doctor), I must mainly rely on the evidence, both for and against from which to draw my conclusions. That necessity, and the data presented in this book, leads me to generalize that the mainstream has the best diagnostic machines, alternative medicines have the most holistic medicines (most compatible with Nature), and GNM has the best answer of cause, which for me, illuminates the best course of action in pursuing the regaining of health.

GNM has only enjoyed the benefit of a small amount of research years, and most of them from a single man, Dr. Hamer, versus the millions of person-years of research behind each of the mainstream and ancient paradigms; there is still much to learn. Its cornerstone is that the psyche while trying to keep you alive, is responsible for most of the situations you call disease. At its core is an understanding that Nature does not make mistakes, and that any conclusion to the contrary is the product of human ignorance. Your task is to dispel this ignorance, to understand why Nature is doing what she is doing, and to do this ideally while you have your health. For me, GNM best answers the question of cause, which I deem crucial in overcoming illness. That its cost is orders of magnitude cheaper than the status quo, is icing on the cake.

Understand that GNM does require full participation in your own health; it is not a spectator sport. View this book as an introduction, not

Conclusion

as a textbook, not as a DIY guide. I strongly advise you consult a doctor experienced in GNM for any medical issue that you might have, should you want to explore this paradigm-shifting therapeutic modality further.

I will now take advantage of a curious cultural phenomenon to complement my conclusion. Often, we are presented with private details of the lives and deaths of public figures merely by consuming the news. I confess to a morbid fascination with post hoc diagnosis using my evolving understanding of GNM. Naturally, we receive this information thirdhand, so this little exercise can only be anecdotal, as important particulars are understandably scant. As such, I will necessarily paint with broad strokes over various celebrity afflictions, and leave it to you to decide the plausibility of my analyses.

Steve Jobs, CEO Apple Inc. Reported to have died of pancreatic cancer. Quote[275]: "I will spend my last dying breath if I need to, and I will spend every penny of Apple's $40 billion in the bank, to right this wrong," Jobs said. "I'm going to destroy Android, because it's a stolen product. I'm willing to go thermonuclear war on this." The cause of his cancer was not made clear by the press.

My analysis using GNM: The pancreas has three functions that respond to three different conflicts: territorial-anger (battles with Microsoft, which he claimed *stole* the MacOS interface for Windows, and Google, which he claimed *stole* the IOS interface for Android), indigestible-morsel (was unsuccessful in stopping either *theft*), and resistance (fired from the company he founded in the mid 1980s). Mr. Jobs was a passionate man, one who had a reputation for confrontation.

Bob Marley, musician. Reported to have died from melanoma. The initial site of the cancer was his big toe, which was said to have been repeatedly injured over several years from playing street soccer.[276] His doctors reportedly attributed his cancer to genetic factors.

My analysis using GNM: The corium skin reacts to attack conflicts by thickening or growing flat tumors, to better protect. It is easy to see how surgical efforts to remove these growths could be perceived as yet another attack, leading to a *spreading* of the tumor.

Gilda Radner, comic, actress. Reported to have died from ovarian cancer. She tried unsuccessfully to conceive with her husband, Gene Wilder. After undergoing fertility treatments, she suffered two miscarriages before being diagnosed with ovarian cancer.[277]

My analysis using GNM: The loss of a loved one (in this case the miscarried fetuses), can trigger the ovaries to undergo necrosis. After the conflict is resolved, the necrosis is reversed, forming cysts (diagnosed by oncologists as ovarian cancer), which fill with mesodermal hormone-producing (estrogen) tissue. The increase in estrogen has the effect of making the woman look younger (smooth skin, glow), while increasing her readiness to mate.

In a male, a similar process occurs in the testicles, albeit with male hormones, which was the event that inspired Dr. Hamer to discover the First Biological Law of German New Medicine, the Iron Rule of Cancer.

Lynn Redgrave, actress. Reported to have died from breast cancer. A large lump was found in her right breast in 2002.[278] As she was right-handed, GNM would predict trouble with spouse (not children or mother). In 1998 she allegedly learned her husband fathered a child with her personal assistant, who later married their son in 1994.[279]

My analysis using GNM: The breast reacts to 2 different conflict shocks: nest worry, affecting the breast glands (this child was raised as her grandson), separation, affecting the milk ducts (as in wanting to separate from her husband).

Bobby Fischer, world chess champion. Reported to have died from kidney failure. Although married to a Japanese national, Mr. Fischer

Conclusion

lived his final years in isolation in Iceland,[280] having close contact only with the family (wife and two children) of his best friend. In 2004, Iceland agreed to offer asylum to Mr. Fischer who was fighting extradition to the United States, his homeland.

My analysis using GNM: Conflicts that affect the kidneys play a huge role in GNM. The kidney collecting tubules are affected by abandonment conflicts (Mr, Fischer was world famous, yet, in the end, saw only four people, two adults, regularly), existence conflicts (poor prognosis from his doctors), and refugee conflicts (could not return to his homeland for fear of incarceration), all of which can be inferred from Mr. Fischer's circumstances. Also, the kidneys are affected by fluid conflicts, which can manifest abstractly as money problems.[281] Conflicts of this sort can eventually lead to renal failure if not resolved.

George Harrison, musician. Reported to have died from multiple cancers, including lung. Mr. Harrison had previously survived a knife attack in which he was stabbed ten times in the chest.[282] His doctors attributed his lung cancer to smoking.

My analysis using GNM: The lungs react to three different conflict shocks: death-fright, affecting the alveoli (after his attack, Mr. Harrison is reported to have said he thought he was going to die), territorial-fear, affecting the bronchials (the attack occurred in his house), and attack, affecting the pleura (for which stabbing certainly qualifies).

Joe Paterno, college football coach. Reported to have died from lung cancer, two and a half months after a child sex abuse scandal involving a trusted member of his staff broke in the news.[283]

My analysis using GNM: As above, the lungs react to three different conflict shocks: death-fright, affecting the alveoli (Mr. Paterno was an 85-year-old devout Catholic. Did he fear having to answer to God for his involvement in the scandal?), territorial-fear, affecting the bronchials (legacy, job), and attack, affecting the pleura (which Mr. Paterno experienced in the media as the direct supervisor of the suspect).

Tony Gwynn, hall-of-fame baseball player. Reported to have died from salivary gland cancer.[284] Speculation centered on his use of chewing tobacco, which carries on it a warning: "This product may cause mouth cancer".

My analysis using GNM: The salivary glands produce saliva, to better lubricate the (food) morsel so that it can be swallowed or spit out. He is reported to have used up to two cans per day for 31 years. That would place enormous stress on the salivary glands to keep up, which, with a DHS, would result in augmentation of saliva producing cells (extracellular growth for an extended period naturally produces a lump, a tumor). What this DHS could have been was not reported.

Ray Charles, musician. Lost his eyesight as a child after witnessing his younger brother's drowning.

My analysis using GNM: If the movie *Ray* accurately portrayed the drowning in question,[285] then not only did the young Ray witness the event, but he was partially blamed for the death by his mother for not alerting her in time. The movie portrayed a textbook example of a DHS. It is easy to imagine the resulting SBS removing his sight, shielding him from further such shocks. Because he was never exonerated, the conflict never resolved, and his SBS never moved to phase 2, reversing the cell loss and restoring his lost eyesight.

Ultimately, it is your health that is at stake. Whether you believe that balancing your energies, or your skeleton, simply hydrating yourself or cutting out parts of your body your surgeon deems superfluous or decayed, ingesting Nature's pharmaceuticals, or patented ones, or attempting to understand your psyche's role in illness, you should honestly embrace it.

Extras

This chapter is home to phenomena that don't fit into the other sections of this book. They do not belong to category F; indeed they are not diseases at all, and are as such, poorly served by most medical paradigms. Their presence in this world is devastating and yet remains for the most part unexplained by conventional authority, a fact which in itself is a source of discord. Because of this silence, I feel obliged to include the following studies, not to distress those already affected, as I have no desire or reason to add to their pain, but to alert those who might still be affected, of compelling evidence as to cause.

Down Syndrome

Down syndrome (DS) is a condition that some people are born with, where it appears that something has interfered with fetal development. People with DS typically have a small stature, low muscle tone, and a sweet, childlike disposition. Mainstream medicine has identified an extra copy of chromosome 21 in people with Down syndrome, which is blamed for the condition. In typical allopathic style, quite a bit of work has gone into identifying three distinct types of DS: trisomy 21 (nondisjunction), translocation and mosaicism. Why the extra chromosome is present, however, is still unclear, and a cure is barely even imagined. Conventional wisdom suggests that as women age, their eggs become genetically less viable, leading to errors in cell division which result in higher incidences of DS. In this view, Nature has once again failed.

GNM offers an explanation[286] via a question. If the fetus experienced a DHS, how would that happen? Sight? No, there is very little light in a womb. Smell? No, the fetus is floating in amniotic fluid; your sniffer doesn't work too well underwater. Taste? No, for the same reason as smell. Touch? Doubt it, as the fluid in the amniotic sac protects the fetus from outside contact. Sound? Bingo! Sound travels very well through water, which actually acts as an amplifier. Products that mimic the familiar sounds of the womb (mother's heartbeat, white noise [to approximate muffled background noises], etc.) are actually marketed to soothe newborns. How might a fetus react to strange loud external noises? Since every other DHS is subjective, there is no reason to believe that a DHS experienced during gestation is otherwise.

We generally treat sudden, loud, unknown sounds with at least caution. Often they are startling, even shocking. Usually, our initial shock quickly gives way to recognition and calm, as we realize the sound poses no danger. The fetus has no such advantage. We cannot reasonably expect it to understand the source of the noise, and the mother has no way of reassuring her unborn child. How does a fetus interpret blaring music, loud street sounds, screeching saws, cacophonous machine noises, etc.? Can some develop a DHS from such exposure? I really don't see how they could not, as it is easy to see how all the conditions for a DHS are readily met. From there, it is not such a big leap to entertain the idea that these conflict shocks might disturb or even interrupt fetal development. Might such disturbances result in Down syndrome?

How is ultrasound perceived in the womb? This is a disturbing question, involving the allopathic compulsion to measure, to see (x-rays, CT scans, EEG, EKG, PET scans, MRI scans, etc.) Can a fetus actually hear ultrasound? The main ultrasound frequency of 2.5 MHz, lies well outside of human audio frequency range (20 Hz to 20 kHz), but are

Conclusion

secondary vibrations caused by ultrasound? Medical researchers say yes,[287] and the sound, which they describe as similar to high notes on a piano, is not subtle; 100 dB (equivalent to a subway train entering a station) was recorded by pointing the ultrasound probe directly at the microphone. Could that trigger a fetal DHS? Consider, that as a woman ages, pregnancies are more closely monitored. How? Well, with ultrasound. The older the mother, the more frequently the child is monitored. Could that fact, rather than a failure of Nature, have something to do with the startling increase in the risk[288] of DS in older mothers?

I am happy to report the good news that GNM has had some success[289] in mitigating, if not reversing, the symptoms of Down syndrome. Much research is still needed, but the initial results are encouraging.

Sudden Infant Death Syndrome

SIDS is defined[290] as the unexplained death of an otherwise healthy sleeping infant. Admitting that the cause of SIDS is unknown, experts in the field suspect defects in, or problems with, the breathing control center of the brain.

Several factors are identified by mainstream medicine as complicit in SIDS, such as sex, age, and race of the child, family history, exposure to tobacco smoke, and being born prematurely. Why these factors should contribute to SIDS is unclear; they seem to be statistical observations. Also associated with SIDS is respiratory infection, as apparently many of the victims had recently experienced a cold.

How is SIDS explained by GNM? I can find no mention of the event in my collection of Dr. Hamer's writings, but taking clues from mainstream speculation (brain issues), an EC complication is immediately suspect. The second phase of any SBS (2-phase reaction to conflict shock) includes a brief return to ST (patient is alert) known as the epileptoid crisis (EC). Recall that all DHSs affect the psyche, brain and organ simultaneously. During healing, in the EC, fluid (all cellular repair takes place in a fluid medium) is expelled from the affected organ as well as from the brain in the location of the HH (concentric ring pattern). This is natural, and normally not a problem, but if extra fluid is present, from a KCT SBS (see *Kidney and Bladder* chapter), there will likely be more pressure exerted by the EC on the surrounding tissues, which could possibly disrupt nerve signals near the HH. If these nerves control breathing (respiratory infection indicates a lung SBS in PCL [healing phase]), then a possible explanation for SIDS emerges. This scenario is not specific to any given age, but I suspect that babies are more susceptible to its complications.

The kidneys, or more specifically, the kidney collecting tubules (KCT), react to conflicts of abandonment, existence, hospitalization, refugee, and isolation. How might an infant experience such a DHS, thereby implicating KCTS in SIDS? Since I am not a trained medical researcher, I can only speculate, and hope for a formal investigation, as the current non-answers ("unexplained" and "unknown") to this catastrophic misfortune are unacceptable.

These conditions, as well as the diseases explored in earlier chapters, evoke strong emotions in those whose lives have been so touched. It is not my intent to stoke those flames. I desire only that the suffering end, a goal which I believe is best achieved with knowledge of cause. Palliative care is by comparison a pale substitute.

Final Thoughts

It is relatively easy to find problems with medical theories, usually, none so much as the status quo, as entrenched interests, agendas, and politics often accompany their existence. Solving those problems by proposing new solutions is a much more difficult task. Without acknowledgment of the problem(s) however, I fail to see why that exploration would ever begin. I believe we have a moral duty to the truth, no more so than with regard to our health. Blind acceptance, as fact, of conventional dogmas riddled with so many open questions, is a dangerous, and historically fatal trap.

My embrace of GNM was heavily influenced by my lifelong gut feeling that Nature (or God if you prefer) is not flawed and mistake-prone. To fully embrace many medical modalities, you have to believe that she is. To me, that has always been a major disconnect. How else though, are what appear to be senseless breakdowns in human health to be explained? The five biological laws of GNM elegantly bridge that gap for me. They offer rational explanations of health issues that do not demand I accept that Nature has failed. Quite the contrary; these symptoms now make sense to me. I don't like them any better than I did, but understanding cause breeds confidence that I will prevail.

Having had pets, I was comforted by observing that when they got sick, that Nature somehow had their backs, that they were listening to her, following her lead to get well again. Call it instinct, but they listen. I don't think we do anymore; I don't think we know how anymore. We

Final Thoughts

seem to have lost an important part of what connects us to a core part of this world. GNM is helping me rediscover it.

In conclusion, as a society, we have the health care we allow. Frederick Douglass wrote: "Power concedes nothing without a demand. It never did and it never will. Find out just what any people will quietly submit to, and you have found out the exact measure of injustice and wrong which will be imposed upon them, and these will continue till they are resisted with either words or blows or both. The limits of tyrants are prescribed by the endurance of those whom they oppress."

The power he was speaking of was government, but make no mistake, the political power the healthcare industry (especially the mainstream) wields is considerable. You are made aware of it through forced vaccinations, the overriding of parental decisions in the care of minors, and now, mandatory insurance participation. Is that where it ends, or is this just the tip of the spear? Unless the status quo is omniscient, a claim which is not made, and one which I feel justified in dismissing, then it too is subject to error, often great error, which we must be free to question and resist.

No field currently commanding 1/6 of the GDP of the United States, and a similar percentage of the output of the rest of the world, operates devoid of politics.[291] Such influence is naturally and understandably used for the benefit of the organization that commands it. Those who avail themselves of mainstream medical services are fortunate if their interests coincide. It too will yield nothing without a demand, which, if you feel is justified, must come from all of you. I do not see how blows are of any use in this struggle; words and choice are my preferred tools. If you say stay silent, if you continue to meekly participate in what you perceive to be a system in need of a course correction, if you make no demand, nothing will change – it will have no incentive to do so.

Reference

German Language GNM Resources

- Dr. Ryke Geerd Hamer website (https://goo.gl/kWGiDw or http://www.drrykegeerdhamer.com/de/index.php)
- Harald Baumann website (https://goo.gl/JPsPcH or https://www.knautsch.ch/HaraldBaumann.php)
- Helmut Pilar website (https://goo.gl/86FtxK or https://www.germanische-heilkunde.at/startseite.html)
- Andreas Baumeister website (http://www.nm-baumeister.de)
- Extensive German language GNM website (http://www.neue-medizin.de)
- The 5 Biological Natural Laws, 4 hour-long documentary with English and many other language subtitles (http://www.5bn.de)
- GNM book store http://www.geneme.ch/medien.html

English Language GNM Resources
- Scientific Chart of Germanic New Medicine, Dr. Ryke Geerd Hamer, ISBN 978-84-96127-29-6
- The Ultimate Conspiracy, James McCumiskey, ISBN 978-0-7552-1470-9
- The New Medicine, Lars Peter Kronlob, ISBN 978-3-936830-53-8
- Ilsedora Laker website (http://www.newmedicine.ca)
- Caroline Markolin website (http://learninggnm.com/home.html)
- Neal Smookler website (http://www.newmedicineonline.com)
- No fear of Cancer, 50 minute interview https://goo.gl/REYstU or https://www.youtube.com/watch?v=bgkZ3Iuff3o

- Biogeneology (GNM related medical paradigm)
    - The Biogeneology Sourcebook, Christian Flèche, ISBN 978-1-59477-206-1
    - Biogeneology, Patrick Obissier, ISBN 978-1-59477-089-0

Nutrition Resources
- Weston Price Foundation website (https://www.westonaprice.org)
- Nourishing Traditions, Sally Fallon, ISBN 978-0967089737
- Fresh Vegetable and Fruit Juices, N.W.Walker, ISBN 0-89019-06704

Other Resources
- The Persecution and Trial of Gaston Naessens, Christopher Bird, ISBN 0-915811-30-8
- Fear Of The Invisible, Janine Roberts, ISBN 978-0955917721
- The Dream and Lie of Louis Pasteur, R.B.Pearson, ISBN 0-646-19541-7
- Functional Processes of Disease, Robert H. Walker http://www.healthresearchbooks.com

Appendix

US Federal spending[292] (millions) on diseases covered in this book

Research	2013	2014	2015	2016	2017(est)	2018(est)
Allergies						
Hay Fever	$9	$6	$5	$7	$7	$5
Food Allergies	$36	$35	$39	$76	$78	$59
Total	**$45**	**$41**	**$44**	**$83**	**$85**	**$64**
Bones and Cartilage						
Arthritis	$231	$239	$214	$248	$256	$193
Dental Disease	$480	$483	$493	$518	$537	$407
Osteoarthritis			$76	$76	$79	$60
Osteogenesis Imperfecta	$8	$11	$11	$16	$16	$12
Osteoporosis	$164	$141	$146	$141	$146	$111
Rheumatoid Arthritis			$59	$91	$94	$71
Total	**$875**	**$863**	**$929**	**$983**	**$1128**	**$854**
Brain						
Acquired Cognitive Impairment			$798	$1132	$1134	$891
Brain Disorders	$3708	$3894	$3916	$4577	$4571	$3640
Cerebral Palsy	$18	$21	$20	$26	$26	$20
Dementia	$650	$704	$721	$1054	$1055	$829
Frontotemporal Dementia	$32	$37	$36	$65	$65	$52
Headaches	$25	$24	$24	$24	$25	$20

Appendix

Huntington's Disease	$55	$50	$39	$37	$37	$30
Migraines	$19	$20	$20	$18	$18	$14
Sleep Research	$229	$233	$313	$315	$316	$254
Stroke	$282	$300	$288	$308	$307	$246
Vascular Cognitive Impairment/Dementia		$45	$72	$89	$89	$70
Total	**$5018**	**$5328**	**$6247**	**$7645**	**$7643**	**$6066**

Research	2013	2014	2015	2016	2017(est)	2018(est)
Cancer						
Cancer	$5274	$5392	$5389	$5589	$6032	$4696
Cancer Genomics				$861	$931	$728
Total	**$5274**	**$5392**	**$5389**	**$6450**	**$6963**	**$5424**

Central Nervous System						
ALS	$39	$48	$49	$52	$55	$42
Alzheimer's Disease	$504	$562	$589	$929	$1348	$790
AD Related Dementias			$120	$175	$234	$146
Huntington's Disease	$55	$50	$39	$37	$39	$30
Multiple Sclerosis	$112	$102	$94	$97	$101	$77
Parkinson's Disease	$135	$139	$146	$161	$169	$129
Total	**$845**	**$901**	**$1037**	**$1451**	**$1946**	**$1214**

Heart						
Atherosclerosis	$374	$375	$386	$385	$397	$309
Cardiovascular	$1964	$1950	$1991	$2108	$2169	$1701
Chronic Obstructive Pulmonary Disease	$102	$107	$97	$97	$100	$79

Appendix

Congenital Heart Disease				$111	$114	$90
Heart Disease	$1230	$1224	$1262	$1289	$1326	$1042
Hypertension	$222	$216	$214	$224	$230	$179
Pediatric Cardiomyopathy				$27	$28	$22
Total	**$3892**	**$3872**	**$3950**	**$4214**	**$4364**	**$3422**

Research	2013	2014	2015	2016	2017(est)	2018(est)
Kidneys and Bladder						
Interstitial Cystitis	$10	$9	$10	$9	$9	$7
Kidney Disease	$551	$549	$564	$574	$593	$463
Polycystic Kidney Disease	$40	$36	$29	$26	$27	$21
Total	**$591**	**$585**	**$593**	**$600**	**$629**	**$491**

Liver and Gallbladder						
Chronic Liver Disease and Cirrhosis	$282	$293	$295	$293	$304	$233
Digestive Diseases - (Gallbladder)	$10	$9	$8	$11	$12	$9
Liver Disease	$594	$605	$616	$635	$661	$509
Total	**$886**	**$907**	**$919**	**$939**	**$977**	**$751**

Lungs						
Acute Respiratory	$95	$85	$108	$103	$108	$83
Asthma	$207	$241	$281	$266	$275	$200
Cystic Fibrosis	$78	$77	$80	$89	$91	$71
Emphysema	$24	$27	$28	$29	$30	$24
Lung	$1230	$1329	$1619	$1604	$1669	$1305

Appendix

Pneumonia & Flu	$407	$362	$384	$380	$393	$311
Smoking & Health	$321	$320	$298	$298	$314	$245
Tuberculosis	$240	$279	$272	$290	$300	$223
Total	**$2602**	**$2720**	**$3070**	**$3059**	**$3180**	**$2462**

Mental Illness

Anxiety Disorders			$156	$174	$183	$140
Attention Deficit Disorder (ADD)	$49	$44	$41	$47	$50	$35
Bipolar Disorder			$80	$90	$95	$74
Depression	$415	$396	$390	$410	$430	$333
Eating Disorders	$31	$30	$31	$28	$30	$23
Mental Health	$2174	$2213	$2263	$2454	$2570	$1985
Mental Illness				$826	$867	$672
Schizophrenia	$232	$253	$241	$254	$268	$207
Serious Mental Illness		$407	$381	$400	$421	$326
Total	**$2901**	**$3343**	**$3583**	**$4683**	**$4914**	**$3795**

Research	2013	2014	2015	2016	2017(est)	2018(est)

Pancreas

Diabetes	$1007	$1011	$1010	$1084	$1105	$951
Total	**$1007**	**$1011**	**$1010**	**$1084**	**$1105**	**$951**

Skin

Psoriasis	$12	$13	$14	$18	$18	$14
Small Pox	$30	$24	$17	$49	$51	$38
Total	**$42**	**$37**	**$31**	**$67**	**$69**	**$52**

Grand Total	**$23,978**	**$25,000**	**$26,802**	**$31,258**	**$33,003**	**$25,546**

Index

2-Phase	46,48,55,74,83,106,132,147,156,193

A

Abstraction	51,85,127,163,172
Acid Test	14
Acne	54,174
AIDS	11,25,40,65-66,140,143
Alcoholism	135,154-155,157
Allopathy	35,37,42,73-74,79,89,91,93,95-96,
	102,111,117,119,136-137,140,144,
	146,155,162,169-174

ALS	93,114-119
Alternative Medicine	43,53,59,76,104,112,141,180,184-185
Alzheimer's Disease	9-10,88,90-91
Antibody	72,137-139
Antoine Béchamp	21-22,32,52
Anxiety	12,54,104,153-154,156-158
Arrogant	13,146
Artifact	46,50,109
Arthritis	77,79,84-85
Asthma	92,144,146,149
Atherosclerosis	89-90,92,120,123
Athlete's Foot	54,169,174
Attack Conflict	57,64-65,106,111,171-175,187
Authority	13,165,190
Ayurveda	39,63,103,125
Axiom	2-3,24,73,137,180,183

B

Bacteria	17-18,24-25,32-33,80,85,106,
	133,136,145-149,164,169-174

Bedwetting	133
Biological Law	45,48,51,60,1105,148,187
Biological Advantage	58,128,155
Bird, Christopher	34,197
Blue Socks	38
Brain	16-19,33,38,46,48,50-58,60,67,75, 87-94,99,102,109,114,116,122-127, 132,153,155-159,171,192-193
Brain Tumor	92,94,102,109
Brainstem	56-57,106,108-109,132,149-150,163
Brain Map	50
Brendan Stack	82
Bronchitis	66,144,147-148
Bubonic Plague	64

C

Cancer	5,10,15,31,38,48,95-113,142,247
CDC	28
Cerebellum	57,106-107,149,157-158,172
Cerebral Medulla	57-58,126,133
Cerebral Cortex	58,108,156,163-164
Chicken	16
Chiropractic	43,74,81
Cholesterol	121-122,127-128
Cognitive Dissonance	3
Common Cold	14,54,148
Concentric Rings	46,50
Conflict-Active (CA) Phase	46,60,75,83,92,107,132,142,149,172
Conflict Resolution	47-48,52,60-61,63-64,85,92, 106-107,117,126-128,134, 148,164,171-172,184
Conflict Shock	45-52,57,60,63,74,83-84,92,106-108, 118,128,132,142,147, 149-150,156,

203

Index

	159,166,184,191,193
Constellation	155-159
Consumption	149
CT Scan	46,50,92,106,109,128,156,159,167, 184,191
Cure	11-13,45,59,91,116,119,134,146,184
Cystic Fibrosis	144,146-147,149

D

Dementia	87-88,90-91,93-94
Dental Health	78,80,85
Depression	154,157-159
DHS	46,48-58,64,75,83-84,92-93,106-110, 117-119,125,132,147-150,166, 172-173,189,191-193
Diabetes	131,134,161-162,166,178
Dialysis	130,134,178
Diarrhea	66,75
DNA	17,37-38,173
Doctor	iv,1-2,11-15,24,36-37,43,54,67,80-83, 97,107-109,116,133,170,183-184
Doctor B	44
Dosha	39
Down Syndrome	190-192
Drowning	5,149,157,189
Drugs	9,12,35,59-60,67,74,80-81,88,91,101, 112,116,124,136,143,155,184

E

Eating Disorders	153-154,157
EC	47,61,92,118,126,133,148,155
EECP	124
Ehrlich, Paul	137

ELISA	137-139
Embryology	16,56,108,132,171,175
Emergency Room	35-36,84,129,134
Ectoderm	56-58,132,141,163
Endoderm	56-57,132,141,163
Evolution	17,48,51,56-57,105,110,132,163,165

F

Facts	2-3,21,23,28,30,38,51,62,64-65,67, 80,84-85,102,112,122,129,136-137, 147,166,170,190,192
Fate	13-15,151
Fear	11-12,19,65,104,110,113,150,188
Ferment	21,32,83
Festinger, Leon	3
Fetus	16,29-30,56,149-150,187,191
Fight or Flight	60,104
Flu	63-66,144-145,148
Fluoride	80-81
Frédéric Bastiat	183
Fungus	33,169,171,174

G

GDP	4,195
Germ Theory	21,24,28,62-64,68,76,137,139-140
Germs	21-24,33,37,52,62
Genetics	73-74,90,100,124,162,168,170,174 180
Glomerular Filtration Rate	131
God	49,58,64-65,188
GNM	45-58,60,63,68,72,74,83-85,92,105, 113,117,128,132,143,148,155,185

Index

H

Hair Loss	85,172
Hamer, Ryke Geerd	45-58,66,76,105,110,113,125-126, 132,134,155,157,171,185,187,196
Handedness	52
Hanging Active	93,106,118,163
Hanging Healing	75,84,93,10g,118,127,133,142-143
Hay Fever	75
Heart Attack	92,120-123,126,129,167
Heart Disease	9-10,43,120-125,129
Hepatitis	135-138,142-143,146
Herbs	10,59,68,103,125,143,184
Herpes	140,169,172
HH	46,48,50-51,92,106-107,109,156,193
High Blood Pressure	90,120,123-124,131,133-134
HIV	25,65-66,75,136,140,169-170
Hobbit	22
Homeopathy	2,41-42,59,103-104
Hopelessness	13,104,112,116,119,134
Huntington's Disease	87-88,90,93

I

Iatrogenic	43
Ignorance	12,15,49,53,59,86,100,107,110, 118-119,128,154,158,183,186
Immune System	22,26,60,72-73,76,137-139,146
Infection	18,24,29,33-34,93,133,137, 143-147,175,192-193
Islet Cells	163,165-166
Isolate	24-26,28,79,82,132,136-140

K

Knowledge Base	1,3-4,15

KCTS	94,127,132,142,148,171,193
Koch, Robert	24
Koch's Postulates	24-26,65,145-146

L

Lanka, Stefan	25,28
Large Trauma	9
Laterality	51,126
Leukemia	99,101,111
Leverage	36-37

M

Malaria	38
Malnutrition	9,79,128
Mania	157-158
Masha and Dasha	23
Measles	23,25-26,28-30,63-64,140,168-171
Medical Theory	2-3,23
Melanoma	66,99,173,186
Menopause	78-79,84
Mesoderm	56-57,187
Metastasis	98,102,109-110
Miasma	63
Microbes	21,23-25,30-31,33,40,48,51-52, 55,137,162,172
Microscope	21,25,29,31-32,137
Microzyma	21,32
Midbrain	57,126
Migraine	87,91,93-94
Morsel Conflict	56,75,106,110,141,163
Mother-Child	19,51,84,106,187,189,191-193
MRSA	33
Multiple Sclerosis	93,114-116,118

Index

N

NAET	74
Nature	iii,3,11-15,17,19,33,48-49,53-58,64, 68,73,76,89,93,107,112,118,123, 162,165,170,179,183-185,190,192
Naturopathic	44,63,104
Naessens, Gaston	32-34,52,180,197
Nutrition	108,122,126,128,197

O

Organ Brain	16-17
Osteoporosis	77-79,82-84

P

Panic	16,20,33,53,64,107,112,118,156
Paranoia	156,158
Parkinson's Disease	114,116,118
Parasites	9,38
Pauling, Linus	122-123,128
Pasteur, Louis	21-23,32,62,64,137,197
PCL	47,56,61,75,92,126,132,142,157,171
Peristalsis	57,111,126
Pesticide	27-28
Placebo	41-42,67-68
Pleomorphic	32,52
Pneumonia	65,144-145,148,170,173
Poison	9,26-29,36,41,66,81,109,112, 125,147,150
Polio	25,27-28,93,140
Price, Weston	82,197
Psoriasis	172
Psychic Shock	49,63,141

R

Rabbits	17
Randomized Control Trial	42,68
Rash	52,75
Reid, Daniel P.	34
Rife, Royal	31,180
Roberts, Janine	28,197
Rutherford, Ernest	38

S

SBS	46-53,74,83,93,106,113,119,126,132, 142,147-150,156,171,184,189,193
Sedative	60-61
Self-Devaluation Conflict	57,65,83-84,111,117
Separation Conflict	52,58,63,65,75,93,111,171-172,175
Sickle Cell Anemia	38
Side Effects	41,81,116,159
Smallpox	25,140,169-170,173
Smoking	40,144,147,150,188-189,192
Somatid	31-34,52
Spanish Flu	63
Spectator Sport	13,185
Spinal Cord	16,99,114,116
STD	168,172,175
Stimulant	60-61,154
Stress Hormones	60
Stroke	10,87-94,120-122,167
Subconscious	15-16,19-20,38,48-49,52,105,159, 165,170,173
Subjective	49,54,107-108,132,192
Sympathicotonia	46-47,59,61,193
Symptom relief	8,12,44-45,53,68,82,91,146,156

Index

T

Terrain Theory	21-23,63,68
Territorial Conflict	55,58,63,65-66,75,111,127,133, 141,147-149,157,164,173,186,188
Tourette Syndrome	82
Tracks	52-53,60,66,74-75,92-94,106,143,184
Traditional Chinese Medicine	39,63,103,124-125
Tuberculosis	56-57,63,106,144-146,148-149,173

U

Ultrasound	191-192

V

Vaccine	26-27,29-30,136,140,143,145,148 168-170,175
Vagotonia	46
Virus	24-30,32,65-66,136-140,142-145, 148,169,171,173
Vitamin C	61,122-123,128-129

W

Walker, Robert H.	17,197
Wasp	20
Water Cure	44,91
Western Medicine	1,11,35,37
Wishes	8,162,179
WHO	146
Worldview	1,3

Y

Yeast	32-33
Yin-Yang	39,103,125

Endnote Instructions

I rely on extensive endnotes for augmenting my case in this book. Most of these link to online articles or webpages, as they are free for you to read, and readily available (requiring only a computer with a web browser and internet access). Since the URLs to these resources can often be very long, I have attempted to make referencing them easy. To that end, I provide two equal methods of doing so for your convenience.

Please visit http://www.acriticallookat.com for the easiest way to view my endnotes. There, you will find an endnote text field on the page, with the cursor ready to accept your keyboard input. Simply enter the endnote number (6, 83, 224, etc.), observe the link information, and press (keyboard) return/enter or click the *original* button to accept and view the webpage the endnote references. As these are third party sites over which I have no control, there is some chance this webpage has changed, moved or no longer exists. If so, and what you see does not make sense in the context of the passage to which I attached the endnote, click instead the *wayback* button and browse the calendar year 2017 or early 2018 entries to see what the page looked like when I wrote this book. In addition, URLs in the *Reference* section are also archived at http://web.archive.org.

Most of the endnotes in the last section of this book are seemingly random 6-character character strings. If you append them to the end of the prefix https://goo.gl/, they form a shortened URL. So, for example, from the *Endnotes* section, we see that the first endnote is Unoqy2. The link to endnote 1 is then https://goo.gl/Unoqy2, which the website goo.gl will translate into the original URL. Also, goo.gl is not a monetized service, so there are no ads to watch before you get to the content.

Endnotes
(see instructions on previous page)

[1] Unoqy2
[2] 5RQmaK
[3] oecuQj
[4] b25rdC
[5] 65Hyga
[6] qHBmk9
[7] uDaQfb
[8] GXokC8
[9] L9vKLp
[10] 4CKh6j
[11] 4x7P8u
[12] 2qTNEC
[13] Y1n4Md
[14] 12FzC3
[15] 39VfSQ
[16] HpYSw1
[17] p1ybQU
[18] acSGBW
[19] gv84dU
[20] oW4GFq
[21] 6hRT6J
[22] The Tao of Health, Sex & Longevity, Daniel P. Reid, page 392. ISBN: 0-671-64811-X
[23] The Persecution and Trial of Gaston Naessens, Christopher Bird, page 5 ISBN: 0-915811-30-8
[24] 26vKr5
[25] 4KtFyx
[26] RQcaGT
[27] w1ehMc
[28] egfnrJ
[29] ba72w7

Endnotes

[30] X9VSDW
[31] n45iU5
[32] 3GEaK1
[33] eWSC5T
[34] xpUQb8
[35] dwBujw
[36] 3Mr5cH
[37] 3n3erH
[38] tYggNr
[39] gPUChU
[40] 58mCTX
[41] wFx4Ad
[42] SnqK3D
[43] Yvp8iu
[44] viNjnj
[45] 91sPwZ
[46] FGXbWu
[47] ns4EUX
[48] t8oy2T
[49] EPMA1d
[50] MiDScA
[51] UBehjn
[52] Bx9Zhv
[53] EKX4WE
[54] zY7pBE
[55] AGtvyg
[56] Scientific Chart of Germanic New Medicine, Dr. Ryke Geerd Hamer, page 29 ISBN: 978-84-96127-29-6
[57] aaDqAk
[58] S3nFuw
[59] wRcery
[60] 5VJPwa
[61] L7pmkX

Endnotes

[62] EhrTyD
[63] DF8K9M
[64] Zb7fTF
[65] RX6rMu
[66] aF3Dof
[67] uJHAfd
[68] gR5v3d
[69] g98j2b
[70] F7122z
[71] 8aPtSn
[72] 9172Zi
[73] tps66L
[74] eNSmcu
[75] Wa3bNt
[76] YVPTNV
[77] MDQJn6
[78] fHtoUS
[79] 9VDg78
[80] j4xxVB
[81] opNr2y
[82] RgoGST
[83] 1767YS
[84] hFhJ3h
[85] cHYy9M
[86] upXSVD
[87] o2nepd
[88] eHSnxN
[89] 1KuoEq
[90] vdT9DS
[91] b3572P
[92] aLw9yi
[93] TGfAju
[94] a4SC19

[95] PEFs4F
[96] gghzCs
[97] RG2aPN
[98] uAGYzv
[99] i2t3Xo
[100] eaUg59
[101] eeKT7w
[102] VkX2G4
[103] FP9mmo
[104] 9dFE3f
[105] srxqBH
[106] K3p2F2
[107] zXpWDZ
[108] ujRJ3K
[109] Uurvzz
[110] GwSTwS
[111] Z52cCT
[112] C83jr3
[113] tThUf3
[114] sqaKQV
[115] VtyZkj
[116] vg2jjR
[117] G9EV5y
[118] wDoXif
[119] sTGgMU
[120] ewCkCR
[121] aHLhdM
[122] 12jxZG
[123] MeaUHL
[124] 3QzYqo
[125] xy7EJg
[126] DdiVJE
[127] nXZcGt

Endnotes

[128] Tj1WDL
[129] qZL4vb
[130] 19Kjjj
[131] suCZDy
[132] uza8hb
[133] 8xFc7V
[134] s2acVG
[135] WDps8Y
[136] TVbsjh
[137] s7XH1Z
[138] BVPG95
[139] vSssU3
[140] bFxW6k
[141] hCYD2x
[142] 14BBSz
[143] A48WH1
[144] 1ksgTA
[145] Guwi5D
[146] myhh3e
[147] qHFUmX
[148] QiGDcM
[149] n8YaEL
[150] c1jgZa
[151] keuV6q
[152] na6CMZ
[153] wPY7Zj
[154] GxASNw
[155] HYhqgL
[156] xJhz1q
[157] qZaBRb
[158] UkTiXN
[159] WXEnEM
[160] YPmcEE

[161] WoxpTL
[162] s9M5hQ
[163] FA41nT
[164] Pi5hC7
[165] e3oWcK
[166] iPnvS4
[167] R7NLg7
[168] RP8nTm
[169] D4KaCg
[170] g8ZzhU
[171] uwqvnF
[172] 8BYKLT
[173] bHpDZe
[174] dLBPBE
[175] PEzuGN
[176] 9ZUyxg
[177] A3UiYa
[178] 2PXENh
[179] vrYauf
[180] 59x8G9
[181] ynCyZV
[182] LYrGkk
[183] 2fNiQ6
[184] fYoSN5
[185] i6ukb8
[186] PDioLN
[187] dRckHw
[188] BSLZbq
[189] Scientific Chart of Germanic New Medicine, Dr. Hamer, page 25
[190] gVR2ks
[191] yj7isz
[192] WyCy7i
[193] EWMakm

Endnotes

[194] THwfNs
[195] dve7Xg
[196] obnjnN
[197] MVKRWN
[198] o7LfFg
[199] 6RjPjm
[200] xExwSq
[201] Jitizr
[202] k6hKkG
[203] SVvTQF
[204] UicVWS
[205] VH9B55
[206] kLC8dx
[207] SC4G4c
[208] TLYLYL
[209] msYBpa
[210] ipC8Us
[211] PFzp2T
[212] 6PneCr
[213] QmuTnq
[214] Juerch
[215] d5uQdu
[216] 8jrHvd
[217] PDdZNd
[218] WJURKW
[219] XQ73EN
[220] FDxkPM
[221] 2aXpLT
[222] EqHYPn
[223] eiadzQ
[224] asYdzw
[225] HvMEL4
[226] 9vVVzm

[227] TfbTj1
[228] miHWv9
[229] gnpgky
[230] 45ZLwC
[231] kHqx37
[232] ket8S6
[233] k9UgVZ
[234] utWfTA
[235] 8onBxp
[236] t7fDQw
[237] hYTNBi
[238] p8ksor
[239] tqwbyh
[240] RLr3ZQ
[241] 9bMbw4
[242] F6FqXu
[243] Moe9Ht
[244] nQQ8P5
[245] 8uE6eo
[246] HB7Exi
[247] 1bxmy
[248] Es5fuY
[249] M3Xctc
[250] aybz9o
[251] W7HE25
[252] 7Gh8Pv
[253] MppucC
[254] GPyW71
[255] SWm6KJ
[256] tucsyq
[257] 9zB28Q
[258] 9RECA8
[259] K3ncT3

Endnotes

[260] YTm2yN
[261] Dk91Zf
[262] Pj8DVt
[263] JAHrKC
[264] btn7Kk
[265] 3Qd5oS
[266] ZDSbkW
[267] F8AfEc
[268] iNxf5J
[269] i6e6VN
[270] TiUQ8A
[271] BuEmwG
[272] 3CEAkd
[273] 2yAgUU
[274] 2xjAHb
[275] cTs8jC
[276] d575z5
[277] DWJKuK
[278] vf54J6
[279] dyoiVo
[280] Wqywqm
[281] c3iSgN
[282] jPUyTt
[283] iNm1Lc
[284] dmuojH
[285] GcqmYi
[286] 2fECrJ
[287] 3QKXTZ
[288] et10AV
[289] UrqigB
[290] BiPdjx
[291] JHsT26
[292] ZWmwRK

Made in the USA
Monee, IL
25 October 2021